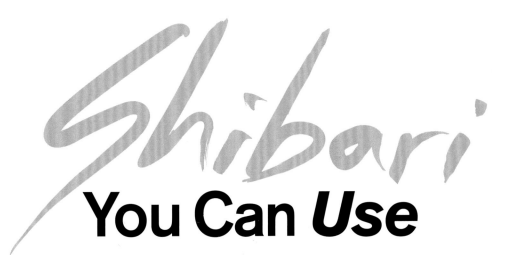

You Can *Use*

Japanese Rope Bondage
and Erotic Macramé

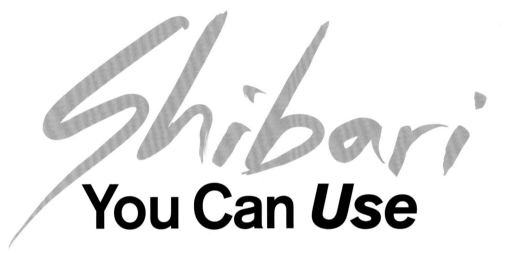

Shibari
You Can *Use*

Japanese Rope Bondage
and Erotic Macramé

By **Lee Harrington**
Photography by **RiggerJay**

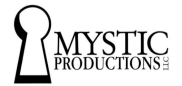

MYSTIC
PRODUCTIONS LLC

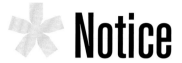 # Notice

Personal responsibility is a basic tenet of adult activity. Like any adult activity, rope bondage inherently contains risk of both physical and emotional injury. Any information or safety guidelines provided in this book are solely suggestions on ways to help reduce those inherent risks. By deciding to engage in any adult activity, including those detailed in this book, you are taking on physical and emotional responsibility for your own actions, and agree to hold harmless all individuals associated with the creation, publication and sale of this book.

All text and rope work by Lee Harrington
www.PassionAndSoul.com

All photography by RiggerJay
www.RiggerJay.com

Book cover and layout design by Rob River
www.RobRiver.com

ISBN 978-0-9778727-2-5
Ebooks: MOBI — ISBN 978-0-9778727-0-1
          ePub — ISBN 978-0-9778727-1-8
          PDF — ISBN 978-0-9778727-8-7

Previously printed in First Edition as ISBN 0-9778727-0-X
and Second Edition as ISBN 978-0-6151-4490-0

Dedicated to our forebearers
who had the courage to
adventure into their passions.

Table of Contents

9   **Introduction**

11   **Chapter One: Background and Basics**
11   Why Bondage?
12   Safety and Negotiation
20   All About Rope
21   The Ends of the Rope
22   Types of Rope
27   Length and Width of Rope
28   Care and Maintenance of Rope

33   **Chapter Two: One-Column Ties**
33   Terminology and Concepts
34   One-Column Tie

37   **Chapter Three: Two-Column Ties**
38   Basic Two-Column Tie
41   Variation: Spread Two-Column Tie

45   **Chapter Four: Shinju (Chest Harnesses)**
46   Basic Chest Harness
51   Clavicle Exposed Chest Harness
53   Adding Rope Option 1: Overhand with Lark's Head
55   Adding Rope Option 2: Lark's Head to Main Body
56   Cupcake Harness
61   Box Tie
67   Halter Top Harness
70   Small Chest Variation
71   Dishevelment

73 Chapter Five: Combinations

74 Gyaku Ebi (Reverse Shrimp)

76 Ebi or Kuri (Shrimp or Ball Tie)

78 Chair Tie

80 Kani (Crab) and Niwatori (Little Chicken)

81 Ankle to Wrist

82 Captive Tie

85 Chapter Six: Rope Corsets and Erotic Macramé

86 Basic Rope Corset

90 Double Spine Rope Corset

94 Fancy Rope Corsets

95 Rope Gauntlets

96 Gauntlet Bondage

97 Chapter Seven: Crotch Ropes

98 Basic Crotch Rope

102 Exposing the Cherry

105 Strap-On Harness

109 Chapter Eight: Where Do We Go From Here?

110 Buy Rope!

112 Get Inspired by More Books

114 Getting Inspired by Other People's Bondage!

116 Practice, Practice, Practice!

117 Acknowledgements

119 About the Author

121 About the Photographer and Collaboration

Introduction

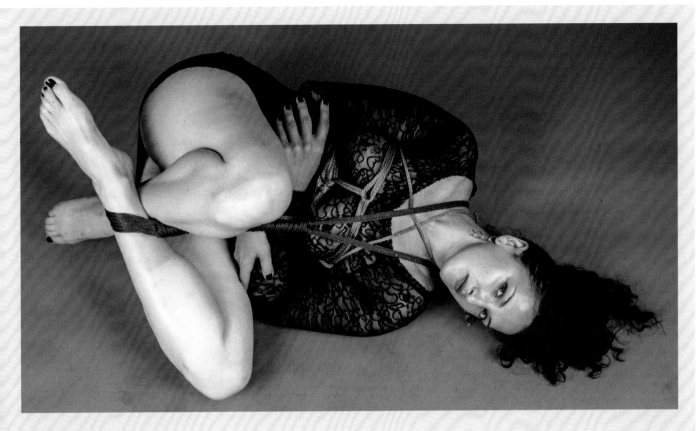

Shall we give it a try?

To begin, we could discuss the origins of rope bondage in the history of feudal Japan and the way it transformed through the ages by way of the theatre into what we know today as Shibari, Kinbaku, or simply but "Japanese Rope Bondage." We could discuss the differences between classical Shibari and Western Shibari, the school of rope bondage into which this book might fall.

But that's probably not why you bought this book.

You want to tie someone up. You want to be tied up. You want to slip this book into someone's hands with a wink and say, "Shall we give it a try?" You want to feel the sensation of rope slipping through your fingers as your lover gasps beneath your bindings. You want to be that bound lover hoping you can stay in rope just a little longer while your partner has their way with you.

That's why you bought this book. Be honest. There is just something about rope bondage that gets people's imaginations going... but when most people look at Japanese-style rope bondage, they are intimidated by the intricacy. They think it takes years of training in far-off dojos to learn even the basics of this mysterious art.

That is a myth.

True, to become a master of any craft you need to dedicate years of study, often under the tutelage of other artisans, and practice regularly. However, to do what most people want to do it only takes a book like this one.

By the end of this book, I'll have taught you enough rope skills that with practice and a patient partner you'll be able to bind someone down to a bed, tie wrist to wrist and ankle to ankle, pull breasts into tight bundles of joy or pain, put your lover into an hogtie or ball-tie, create your own strap-on harness, weave a rope corset... and more.

So pick up this book. Shake off your fears of looking silly the first time you tie someone up, get some rope, and you too can learn Japanese rope bondage and erotic macramé.

This book is not meant for your bookshelf, to gather dust and only be pulled out for titillation value (though feel free to be titillated!). Shibari You Can Use was designed to live in your bedroom, or in a bag of rope and be played with. Pull it out for inspiration before a big date, or blindfold your lover and with this book lying next to them, get rope on them for the first time. Make notes or sketches in the margins if you like, or bookmark your favorite pages!

Have fun, and make this book yours.

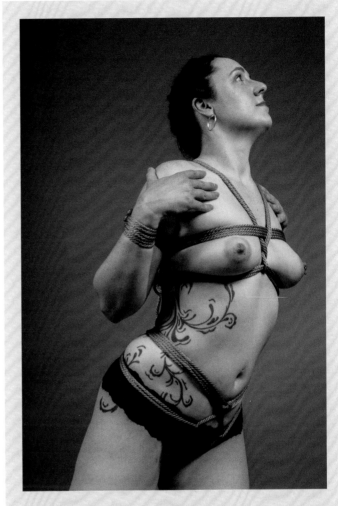

Backgound and Basics

Why Bondage?

Every person I have ever met who does rope bondage as a Rigger/Artist/Top (the person who does the tying) or as a Submissive/Bottom/Model (the person being tied) has a slightly different reason for doing bondage.

A few of those reasons include:

- Restraint
- Meditation
- Inability to escape
- Trance
- Art
- Novelty
- Fetish for rope
- A partner's desire
- Sensuality
- Being silly/playful
- Trust
- Power exchange
- Ritual
- Masturbation
- Consensual torment
- Struggling
- Sex
- Sensation
- Sadism/Masochism
- Exhibitionism/Voyeurism
- Part of role-playing

A Basic Chest Harness (page 46), Crotch Rope (page 98), and Two-Column Ties (page 38) were used to create this simple yet effective tie.

You're not into pain? You can still enjoy bondage. You want to do bondage because you think it's pretty? Fantastic. Is rope bondage a part of your sex life but you don't consider yourself "kinky?" So be it! Being authentic is sexy!

What if you want to experience intense sensations? What if you want to use bondage as part of your spiritual life or to show off your skills in public?

Then do it. Everyone has the right to play with rope!

Safety and Negotiation

Find out what your partner is into

Some folks desire to be tied up because they want to experience intense sensation and pain. Others are interested in doing bondage because it's pretty and they enjoy sensuality. These two folks, if they want to play together, need to negotiate their interests. In fact, it's a great idea for everyone to negotiate!

Find out what your partner is into. Find out what he is not into. Find out if she has limits you need to discuss (some folks don't do sex and bondage, some don't do gags, some don't like to have a submissive role, some want to tie themselves up while you watch... this is a chance to talk about it). Even if their desires are not identical to yours, that is okay. Both partners can take turns having their desires met, or combine their passions into a single scene. Seeing your partner glow can also lead to you feeling your own joy, even if their specific desires are not what you are into.

There are lots of ways to negotiate: tantalizing notes back and forth over email before getting together, formal questionnaires, cuddling up and whispering naughty ideas to each other, or sharing images found online. Find and follow your own personal style for negotiation while remembering that the bulk of communication is non-verbal. "Listen" to what your partner is sharing beyond their words.

Negotiation is not a one-time opportunity to learn about your partner's passions. Each time after you play, you both have the opportunity to debrief with one another about what you enjoyed and what you realized you are not interested in. Continuing the conversation around interest and desire helps the next time be even better.

The continuing conversation around what each of you are into needs to happen internally as well. By playing with rope, you will likely learn what turns you on, and what you want to do more of. Just because you started

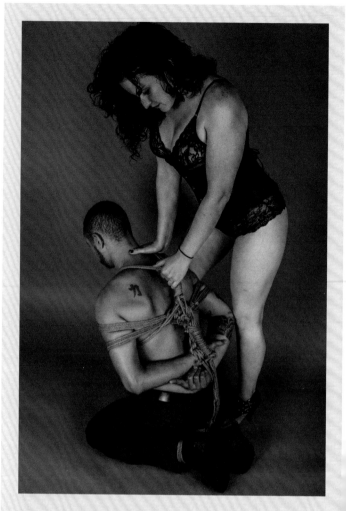

Rope bondage can be a powerful tool for dominance and submission.

your interest in rope bondage because it was beautiful does not mean that you won't delight in bondage where you get a chance to connect with a partner, or have your ropework involve an element of intense sensations. Enjoying these sensations is sometimes referred to by kinky people as sadism and masochism, but should not be confused with the clinical concepts. Kinky masochists and sadists usually want intense emotion and sensation, not to truly cause or receive harm.

Talk about health issues

There are a variety of health challenges that can come into play with rope bondage. Go over them with your partner, and discuss any other possible issues that might be specific to your reality as well. Examples include:

- Allergies (from the grass fibers of hemp rope, to laundry soaps, etc.)
- Asthma
- Diabetes
- Epilepsy or other seizure disorders
- Circulatory or heart problems
- Joint challenges
- Past injuries
- Emotional issues (trauma involving confinement or other triggers)

If any of the above are part of your life, it doesn't mean you can't do rope bondage. It just means be careful. If she has an allergy to hemp, use nylon. If he can't have his hands behind his back because of a torn rotator cuff, tie his hands in front of him or at his sides. If they can't be hogtied because of a bad back, try tying them spread-eagle to a bed. Be creative, work through challenges that may arise, have food nearby for diabetic folks, and have medication nearby for those who need it. Don't let health issues stop you from having fun if you can work around them safely.

These questions apply to Tops (the person doing the binding) just as well as Bottoms (the person being bound). Does your rope Top have health issues you should be aware of? You should also each ask yourselves, "Am I emotionally and energetically okay today?" If either of you is mad, upset, deeply depressed, intoxicated, sleep-deprived, or just in a bad mood, this may not be the time to tie someone up or be tied up.

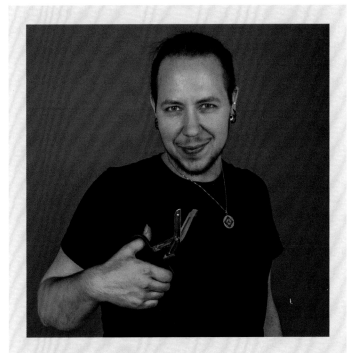

Always keep your safety shears or safety hook handy.

Remember that issues can arise unexpectedly, such as a hip hurting, or breathing becoming restricted. Thus, keeping a watch on your partner is important. This is why doing bondage alone, or leaving the room while a partner is bound, is inappropriate. If something were to come up health-wise, someone else needs to be there to help get them out of the tie.

Places to tie/not to tie

Good ideas: Major muscle groups, torso, forearm, lower leg, thigh

Decent ideas: Back of neck, hands, feet, upper arm (watching out for pressure on nerve bundles), between the legs, around the waist

Bad ideas: Front of neck (choking danger), directly on joints (apply wrist and ankle ties just above the joint)

Be aware that each person's body is slightly different, and as a Bottom, you will come to learn your own body and how it interacts with bondage. If something is tingling, pinching, digging in, hurting or just feels "off"—trust your instincts. Your body awareness is one of the important pieces you bring to a bondage scene, and developing that skill is important.

Tops, this does not negate your responsibility. Checking in with your partner, avoiding body zones that you know are potential health risks, and staying alert and aware during a scene can help keep you and your partner safe. Restraint may look simple and sexy, but simple issues can become big ones, so stay alert. Staying attentive and attuned to your partner also gives you a chance to connect on a deeper emotional level.

Be prepared!

Here are a few things I recommend having on hand before beginning your scene:

Safety Shears/EMT Scissors/Penny Snips: Whatever you call them, get a pair. These are great because they can cut through rope, but have a rounded edge and safety guard so they don't cut skin. Test them out ahead of time and make sure they work. Have them nearby, not buried at the bottom of the drawer or in your bag. If you prefer a seatbelt cutter or other "safety" style knife, those work as well. Sharp blades and knives are discouraged because they are dangerous to use in a dark room under any sort of stressful situation.

Water or other hydrating fluids: People get thirsty being tied up and doing the tying! Consider having a straw for folks tied up to drink through. Caffeinated beverages dehydrate the body, and thus are not what is recommended here.

CPR/First Aid training: Just in case something happens, know how to react and help the situation. Having a phone nearby (on vibrate/silent as to not interfere with your private play and connection time) if an emergency arises is also encouraged.

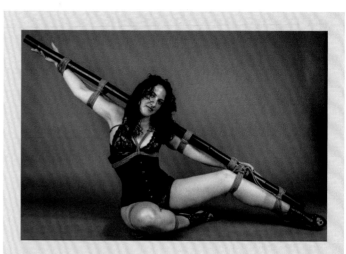

Two-Column Ties (page 38) can be used with bamboo, chairs, and other static objects.

Safewords: Safewords are a tool for folks who like to role-play struggle and "non-consensual" fantasies, or who are involved in power/pain exchanges. Choose a word like "screwdriver" or "banana" that probably won't come up in your play. If either the Bottom or the Top says the "safeword," the scene goes on pause. The players can talk plainly and simply, or decide to have the bondage end right then, depending on what you agree on during your negotiation/discussions in advance. If the Bottom is gagged, have her hold a jingle toy or a colorful scarf. If she drops it, you know there is a problem.

Safewords are only one option for communicating during a scene. Whatever communication style you choose, set your plan in advance for how you will communicate during your play.

Rope: Yup, to do rope bondage, you need rope, or some other material to bind with. Later in this chapter, we will discuss what kind and amount of rope you need. This may sound silly, but I have left my rope in a different room when playing, and had to stop the action to go get it.

Optional Items:

Marlinspike: This blunted spike used by sailors is a good tool to have if your knots tighten up and are hard to untie. You carefully insert the marlinspike into a knot, between the ropes, and wiggle it back and forth until the knot slowly loosens.

Blanket or coat: People can get cold while tied up or after being untied. Having a blanket around is handy. Keeping an "emergency blanket" in your toy bag is useful as well.

Towels: Towels can be used underneath ropes for limbs that have suffered injuries, to place under people if they drool or leak other bodily fluids, or to have on hand for cleaning up spilled drinking water.

External structures: Beds, chairs, tables, ottomans, pillows, eyebolts, etc.—whatever you want to use to tie someone to, tie someone on, or prop someone up with. If the Bottom will be pulling on the structure, like a post on a bed or an eyebolt, make sure it will hold the pressure. Folks who are tied up and struggling can seem to have superhuman strength!

Sex supplies: Dildos, vibrators, condoms, gloves, lube. It's so frustrating if they aren't nearby when you want them. Negotiate for safer sex before you start playing. In fact, some folks don't like combining bondage and sex, or may not be in the mood. Make sure everyone is on the same page before you begin playing, and respect their preferences. Not doing so is not only inappropriate, but may also be a form of abuse due to its non-consensual nature.

BDSM supplies: Blindfolds, gags, nipple clamps, whips, low-temperature candles (for wax play), enema bags, paddles, clothespins. Discuss these things with your Bottom before they are tied up. Consent is key in bondage and other forms of kinky interactions. Kinky play can release endorphins and dopamine, and makes

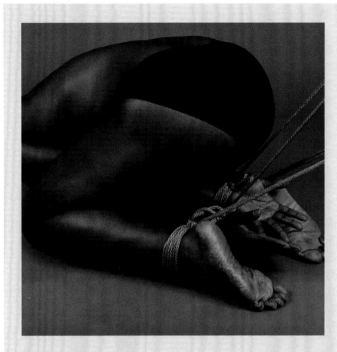

Remember to check for circulation, especially in difficult poses.

renegotiation mid-scene just like trying to renegotiate from other altered states of consciousness. Make sure folks are "sober" when renegotiating.

Wooden dowel or bamboo pole: When doing Two-Column Ties (see page 38), you can use a pole or dowel as one of the columns. Imagine the combinations!

Camera: Some people like to record their bondage (especially if it is intricate). Ask each other in advance if photos or video are desired. Remember, if you want to publish photographs anywhere you will need a model release. If either partner says, "only you get to see the pictures," respect that request. This is especially true for images that might appear online—once something is on the internet, you never really know where it might end up and who might see it.

Encourage stretching

Flexibility is a boon when being tied up. You can hold positions for longer periods, be tied in more challenging poses, and be more comfortable overall. Slow stretches like trying to touch your toes, twisting from side to side, stretching your arms back and various forms of yoga will help keep you from cramping up or having limbs fall asleep as quickly. Also, remember to remove any jewelry that could get in the way of tying such as bracelets, watches, or anklets.

Stretching will not make you able to hold poses forever, and even advanced bondage aficionados can only hold some poses for very short periods of time. There are Bottoms who will be unable to do every position in the book, and there are even harder poses that you will see online—poses almost no one can hold. Make sure to modify your ties to work with the person you are playing with, and don't push your body in stretching or in ties beyond what your body can safely do. Ties can be modified for your body reality.

And while Tops are thinking about it—you should stretch too. It is best to avoid a back spasm mid-scene. While tying, also keep your own body poses in mind. It is easier to tie someone when they are down on the ground if you are sitting right next to them, rather than bending over and straining your back.

Circulation and nerves

Let me preface this material by saying that the author is not a medical professional—please do your own research, and if concerned, make sure to consult with a medical provider.

Blood runs through the body via arteries and veins. When you tighten ropes at various points on the body, you can cut off that blood supply. This leads to limbs changing color, tingling, losing the ability to grip, going cold, and eventually losing sensation.

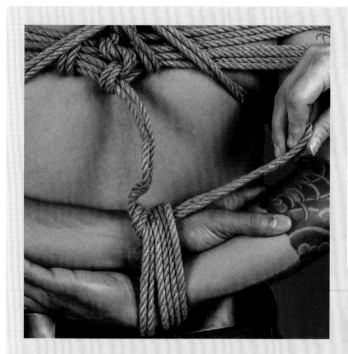

Remember, you can untie someone at any point, even from fancy bondage ties. You can always try again later, or choose a different pose.

If this happens, don't panic.

A good test for circulation begins by squeezing your Bottom's hand before you begin tying. Have him squeeze back. Tell him that any time you squeeze his hand you want him to squeeze back. Periodically, when the Bottom is tied, check his circulation in this manner. If his hand was warm at the beginning but now its ice cold, can he still squeeze? If he can't open and shut his hand at all, or if there are other concerns such as a slow return of color to a limb when pressure is applied to the skin, it is time to move that limb.

Just because you have to move a limb, the scene does not have to be over! Some Bottoms get upset because they feel it is their fault they couldn't hold a pose.

To offset these negative emotions, consider saying something like, "Bwa ha ha, I have a better idea. I want to tie you this way instead." As a Top, you can claim the power to change poses. It's an opportunity for you to try something different with your partner.

The other issue that can arise from rope bondage is nerve impingement. If the Bottom feels tingling, burning electric shock, or other unusual sensations running down their arms (or other limbs)—act immediately. Move the limb, change the rope, or get them calmly out of the tie as soon as you can to avoid the chance of nerve damage.

Bottoms, speak up! If you feel a sharp stab of pain, have a limb fall asleep quickly, or experience tingling sensations, tell the Top. Toughing out any form of nerve challenges is not the course of action to take, especially if your partner does not know you are toughing something out. Even if you are gagged, find a way to communicate these issues, or else your rope bondage scene could lead to serious injury. Three loud grunts allow for a sound from behind a gag, and are unlikely to be confused with any sort of erotic moaning.

Unfortunately, nerve impingement is not always noticeable. Weakness, loss of sensation, and loss of movement (such as "hand drop" when the hand stops being able to hold up its own weight or grip anything) might only come to attention when a scene is done. These signs can affect all or part of the hand (depending on which nerve was pinched), the wrist, the lower arm, and sometimes parts of the legs or feet.

Nerve challenges can arise with tight binding on any areas that press directly into nerves that run close to the surface of the skin. The inside of the armpit, pinky-side of the hand, outside of the upper arm and back of the upper arm have been shown to cause pressure to nerve bundles. Femoral nerves can be challenged by

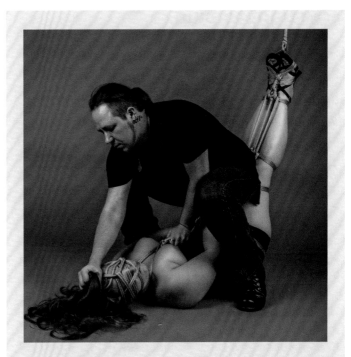

Ask your partner what they like—some people like to have pretty bondage, and others may want to be disheveled.

pressure in the space between the pelvis and upper thigh (in extreme Ebi poses for example), or firm binding around the indent at the top of the thigh. Though this is not an exhaustive list, developing awareness on nerve and circulation systems in the body can be a fun project for people to do together—exploring each other's flesh with your fingers to palpate for the nerve bundles as you build trust and connection. Each person's body is different, so keep that in mind as you play while listening to each other.

If after a scene circulation is overly slow to return, there is a loss of mobility, or pain of any sort caused by the rope or the positions—don't be afraid to see a doctor if problems persist. Most medical professionals are more concerned about getting you healthy than they are about your sexual preferences and predilections.

How tight to bind?

Though it's good to have ropes nice and snug (and lined up flat so as to not dig in unevenly), it is also important to make sure that the rope is not too snug. Try sliding a finger or two under the ropes; if you can't fit one finger between the ropes and the skin, go ahead and loosen the ropes up. Otherwise, it can cut off circulation. With the One-Column Tie, instead of taking the whole cuff off, you can loosen it by releasing the final knot, sliding a finger under, wiggling it looser, and then retying.

As a note though—rope can loosen or tighten on its own. Some rope stretches. Sometimes limbs swell. Sometimes skin gets cold and makes it seem that ropes have loosened. You may rotate or move your Bottom and the ropes move slightly, causing them to loosen or tighten.

Check your ropes from time to time; one to two fingers under the binding is usually good, three to four or more under a tie may be a sign that you need to tighten the bindings if you are trying to restrain their body (rather than decorate it).

Rope marks

Many rope marks are caused by pressure on the skin, and can fade quickly. One exception is what is called a "rope hickey." This occurs when skin gets trapped between two or more pieces of rope and gets pinched between the lines. Capillaries in the skin burst where the skin was pinned leading to lines that are very much like hickeys you give when nibbling on someone's neck. Avoiding minor gaps between adjoining ropes can prevent rope hickeys, but they do happen from time to time to even the most experienced bondage practitioners. Some Bottoms even enjoy them as a badge of honor.

Rough rope is more likely to mark than soft rope. Struggling and tension on rope are more likely to cause rope marks than scenes where the Bottom is peaceful or relaxed. If you are especially concerned

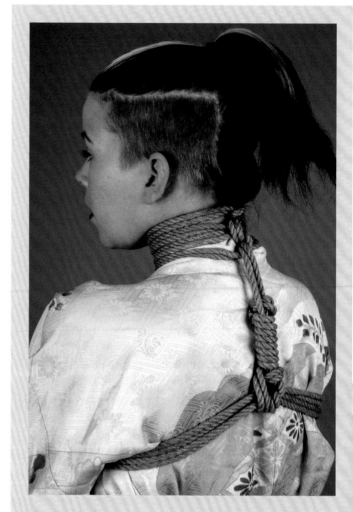

A Basic Rope Corset (page 86) can be used to make an elegant posture collar—but do not tie it very tight.

about marks, consider doing bondage over clothing or other padding, and avoid heavy struggling, as even the most careful rope work occasionally leaves marks on bare skin.

Pulling rope very quickly along the skin can cause what is called "rope burn," a form of mild (or intense) skin abrasion. To avoid it, pull rope slowly, or if going under other ropes, lift up the top ropes and slide the second rope underneath. Rope burns are more likely to happen on dry and cracked skin than on smooth, moisturized skin, so for sensual bondage, consider incorporating massage into your pre-bondage warm up.

Removing rope and post-scene

Don't rush! Feel free to remove ropes slowly, especially if you began the scene by slowly binding your partner. Many people who are new to bondage feel a need to rush out of the ropes when they are done, but part of the joy of rope bondage is the unwrapping process. If you rush out of the ropes, your Bottom may feel disoriented, get frustrated, or have other distress. You also lose a great opportunity for connection and affection. If the bound partner has lost circulation in a limb, there will be a period of pins and needles, so give them time to recover.

Many people also become chilled when released from ropes. Have that blanket or coat handy. Other Bottoms get lightheaded, dizzy, become light sensitive, need food or water, or are on such a "bondage high" that they go silent, act silly, or are not functioning intelligently (let alone capable of driving home safely). Take care of them! If she needs water, get it for her, or better yet, have it there already. Every rope Bottom is different; respect and enjoy their differences.

Listen to their body—and yours! What are your desires in this moment? Do you need a glass of water? Consider tying a wrist cuff on them and have them grab you each a glass of water. This leaves a piece of the rope on their skin, letting them stay connected even as they wander away for a moment. Perhaps you are the one who needs the cuddles. Maybe everyone involved wants to go in for another round of rope play. Make sure all parties speak up for their needs and listen to their personal truths.

Taking care of your partner after a scene does not end 10 minutes after the ropes come off. Hours or even days later, find time to check in with one another.

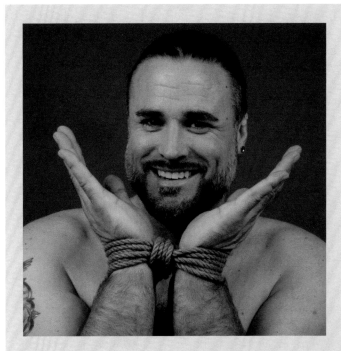

You get to choose whether your play is sensual, solemn, or silly.

Something as simple as an email or phone call can help you connect. This is a chance to find out how your bodies are doing, and get feedback on how to make the scene even better next time.

Some people have emotionally charged reactions to bondage, especially if it was their first time in ropes or their first time playing with you. This experience might feel like falling in love in some cases, so don't make radical life decisions after your first time playing with someone. Tops, as well as Bottoms, may also have "rope drop," an experience where their mood or energy drops after play. Make sure they know you are there to talk with them, or if you are not available, that they have friends who can check in with them. Setting up these back-up folks for additional "aftercare" can be helpful; they're allies for both the Top and Bottom along the process of their kinky journey.

All About Rope

There is no one right rope for rope bondage. Sorry. Each type of rope has its pros and cons. I personally keep a mix of hemp, jute, multifilament polypropylene (MFP), and parachute cord in my toy bag, and occasionally also carry cotton, cheap nylon (for when I know my rope will get trashed in a scene), silk cording or ribbon (for body and head harnesses), and whatever else strikes my fancy.

There is nothing wrong with mixing media; tying someone's hands and chest in polyester then using hemp for everything else is okay, as is being a cotton purist. Read through the list of pros and cons, find sources that allow you to feel each one that sounds good, and buy what works for you. Some people even like combining multiple types of bondage by doing chest harnesses with leather wrist cuffs or rope corsets inside a spandex body sack.

Different individuals will prefer different types of rope. People with a passion for color might choose to buy ropes that match their favorite fetish outfit. Individuals with grass allergies or who have challenges with dust might avoid natural fiber ropes. If sensitivities to laundry soap are a concern, playing with polyester that was washed in such soaps might not be an option.

You might also choose to invest in new ropes due to a specific relationship. There are some couples who will choose to buy a set of rope that is "just theirs," or a Bottom might have rope that only gets used on them. This rope might have an emotional attachment, or because they want their own for hygiene purposes.

This book is for sensual, decorative, floor, and bedroom-based bondage only. I will not be addressing the safety issues for suspension and aerial rope bondage in this book. Don't risk your Bottom's safety by using inappropriate materials or techniques for suspension.

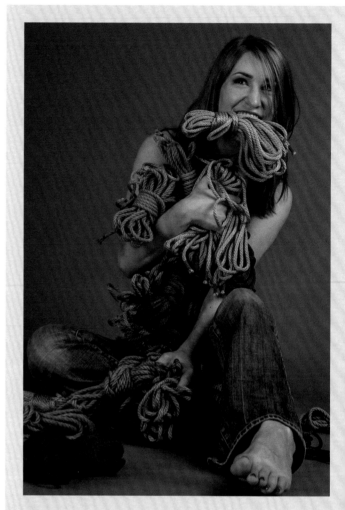

Do you like rope? There are so many different types to experiment with and enjoy!

The Ends of the Rope

There are a wide variety of ways to "finish" the ends of your rope, depending on the material you use and how you like to play. If you do not finish your rope in some way, your rope will begin to unravel, and you might end up with a pile of tangled threads rather than rope you can enjoy.

For a quick and easy start, you can temporarily wrap the ends of your rope tightly in packing tape, duct tape, or a similar material. You might also choose to tie an overhand knot in the ends of your line, producing a bulky finish. Both choices can get you going right now, even if you choose to do something different down the road.

Man-made fibers (such as nylon, MFP and polyester) melt at high heat. Take a lighter or candle and hold the end of your rope over the flame until it melts. Squish the end of the rope to a smooth nub, preferably with something other than your bare fingers (ouch!). Make sure to either file down or smooth the end when melting it to eliminate burrs that could scratch your Bottom when tying him up.

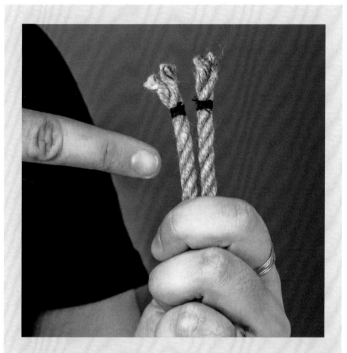

These rope ends are whipped, but play around with different options and use what feels right for you.

The next option is to "whip" the ends of your rope, a technique that involves wrapping thread or a twine around the rope near the end of the line. Whipping the ends of rope can take time, but it leaves the end of the rope soft (for using as a sensation toy) and has a stylish look. Techniques for whipping rope can be found in many knot manuals, home-decorating books or on websites. You can whip almost any type of rope except climbing rope and hard plastic rope.

The last common option is to do knotwork at the end of your rope. Crowned wall knots, Celtic button knots... there are plenty of options. You can even find instructions online for splicing your rope back in on itself to create a useful look for the ends. Knotting can be a good finishing option because you don't have to tie an overhand knot to add on more rope (see page 53). However, end knots can get in the way when you want to quickly go over or under the line, such as when tying chest harnesses.

Types of Rope

Cotton

This is a great option for novices or sensual players: it's soft, has high burn speed (i.e., it takes a lot of pressure/speed to burn the skin), and becomes even softer with washing. It can be very erotic, and you can choose whether you want twisted or braided cotton rope. Cotton is easy to dye to a color you like, or you can give the aesthetic of Western bondage if you leave it white.

A caution: cotton can become fuzzy and dirty, so try to keep it clean. Like all natural fibers, cotton can get hard when wet, making knots difficult to undo, and can become moldy if it stays wet. This rope also stretches a fair bit, with bondage that was snug becoming looser if a Bottom struggles.

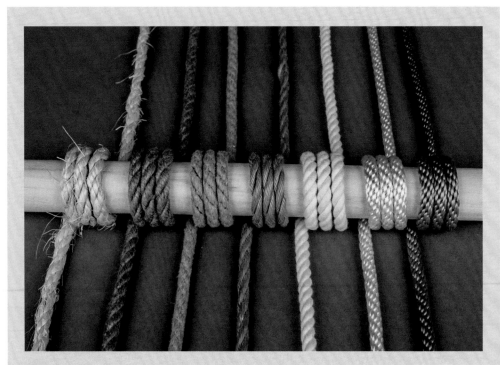

(From left to right) Sisal, Jute, Western Hemp, Japanese Hemp, Cotton, Nylon, Multifilament Polypropylene (MFP)

For those of you living in situations where having lots of kinky toys is tricky, keep your "story" about your rope in mind. It can be hard to explain the 400 feet of custom-dyed jute, but easier to say "this is for hanging clothes" if you have just a few pieces of cotton or MFP. Having a single storage space for your toys is a great option. This applies even if you are free to have your rope anywhere. It lets you know where your rope is for quick access and ease of play.

Climbing Rope

Though rough on the skin, fairly stiff, and quick to burn, this rope will certainly hold up if you're putting a lot of stress on your line. Why? Because that's what it was built to do! It comes in a wide array of colors and patterns, but it can be very pricey and its stiffness makes it challenging to work with in fine detail.

Coir

This natural-fiber rope is made from coconut husks, is very light weight, floats, and is scratchy. Coir also rope burns easily, and is fairly stretchy as far as natural fibers go. If you're a sadist or masochist, this could be the rope for you.

Hemp

Hemp rope is one of the traditional materials for Japanese-style rope bondage, along with jute rope. It is a warm golden color, or with treatment and age, can become a beautiful ash brown. Some folks also dye their hemp rope in myriad colors. Hemp smells like grass or hay, does not stretch much, and holds knots very well. Hemp has a moderate burn speed if treated, but burns quickly if left untreated.

There are different types of hemp rope: twisted tightly (which are firm, sometimes thought of as "Western hemp"), twisted loose (which are soft, but can untwist with some forms of fast tying, sometimes called "Japanese hemp"), and braided hemp. Check which type you are buying, and whether the level of processing and firmness will suit your desires.

If you buy hemp rope in bulk, it comes 100% untreated, is very rough, and often is very light in color. The rope is likely to have splinters in it, and is sometimes uneven in weave. This is good for Bottoms who like painfully intense sensation, but not for many other folks. There are a number of distributors out there who process or dye hemp rope for bondage (see page 110 for resources), as well as "finish" the ends for you (see page 21 for examples). It is possible to treat hemp rope yourself and, though time consuming, many rope artists enjoy the process because they emotionally bond with their rope.

Here's my process for treating hemp rope:

Get a huge pot. Fill it with water and set it to boil. Cut the rope into the lengths you want and tie tight overhand knots at each end to keep it from fraying. Throw the rope in the pot, and let it boil for an hour while stirring regularly. Strain. Squeeze excess water off of the rope, and drape over a pole or drying rack in big loops, with pressure (such as a second pole) on the bottom of the loops to keep tension on the rope. Let it dry for a few days.

Once the rope is completely dry, clear a large open area, remove fire hazards and set up a candle or other small fire source. From one end to the other, run the rope through the flame while rotating or twisting the rope. This will singe splinters or rough spots off the rope. Don't stop moving or you will burn the rope itself. This can be a slow, boring process; put on some good music and stay focused on the project.

Lastly, find a piece of heavy canvas, or, if you are the hands-on type, use your hands for this step. Put a small

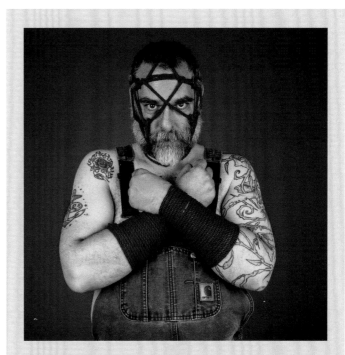

A masculine look can be created with a Head Harness (*More Shibari You Can Use*) and Rope Gauntlets (page 95).

dab of hemp oil or mink oil on the cloth or your hand, and slowly pull the rope through the cloth from one end to the other. This small amount of oil will allow the rope to slide more smoothly across the skin.

You don't need much. Then run your hand back over it again and make sure it looks and feels even and has no big globs of oil anywhere. Beeswax is also a good tool to consider. Hang your rope up to dry again—voilà!—you've treated your rope.

Though hemp is technically machine washable (see page 28), machine washing can untwist hemp, remove natural oils, or break down the strength of hemp over time. Some people prefer to boil their rope after it has been exposed to bodily fluids, but it's your choice. If you choose to wash or boil your rope, consider re-oiling it from time to time to keep it soft and supple.

Jute

Another natural fiber like hemp, jute has more of a licorice smell than a grass smell. There are some Riggers who have developed a strong passion for jute over hemp, while others are happy to play with either. It has a deeper golden brown to it, and is a favorite of many erotic photographers for the rope patterns it leaves on the skin and its "classical" appearance.

Jute expands when it gets wet, more so than hemp, so think twice before throwing a bound Bottom in the bathtub unless you have a pair of shears or a marlinspike nearby. This rope has a burn factor slightly higher than that of hemp, but that friction can also be used as a delightful sensation toy during play. It holds knots very well, but when it is first being used, it can creak a bit. Jute can be processed in the same manner as hemp if desired, and many fine retailers carry a variety of jute rope.

Nylon

Cheap, widely available, and popular, this smooth and silky rope is flexible and soft on the hands and body. However, it does stretch (though not quite as much as cotton), and has a low burn speed. Nylon is perfect for slow romantic or sensual scenes, even with a bit of struggling. Unfortunately, due to its silkiness, nylon does not hold a knot as well as natural fibers. Sometimes it will be necessary to tie an additional hitch after all your bondage work is done, just to make sure the rope doesn't slip.

A great bonus? Nylon does not expand when it gets wet, and thus is wonderful for using on sweaty Bottoms or in the shower. Nylon comes in three major varieties: solid braid, hollow (or cored), and twisted. Solid braid is nylon all the way through, in the same material, in a single weave of material. Hollow braid is a braided sheath of nylon over a core of another material—sometimes nylon, sometimes monofilament propylene, sometimes multifilament propylene. I like to call hollow rope "mystery rope" because you have no idea what is

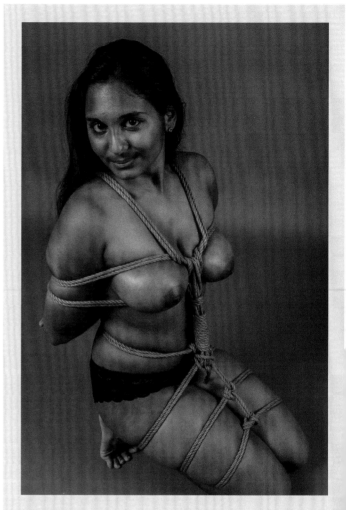

Once you have the basics down, try to create unusual variations, such as this combination made from jute rope.

going on inside the rope—whether internal strands have broken, if your rope is moldy, etc. I recommend against using hollow braid unless it's a spur-of-the-moment scene. The third variety is twisted nylon rope, which is usually three to six strands of nylon (each made of up to a hundred threads) twisted together to form a single rope.

Parachute Cord or Para-Cord

Available in a wide variety of colors, this fine line is perfect for detailed binding, like gently tying a one-column tie around the cock and balls, lashing fingers to one another, or doing intricate knotwork on breasts. Parachute cord has a nylon sheath and a filler core of some sort, varying by brand. If wanting something sturdy and durable, "550 Cord" is the traditional cord of choice for actually jumping out of airplanes, since not everything called parachute cord is actually cord for parachutes. You can either choose to work with para-cord as is, or you can remove the core for a line that will lay flatter against the skin.

Polyester

Often used for macramé in the 1970s, polyester ranges in firmness from stiff and rough to silky smooth. Available in solid braid, hollow braid and twisted, it comes in a diverse palate of colors, and competes with nylon and MFP as an option for bondage, especially decorative rope work. Purchasing your polyester from a bondage vendor makes it far more likely to be of the softer and silkier variety than buying it at a local hardware store.

Polypropylene (MFP)

There are two major types of polypropylene rope—multifilament polypropylene, and monofilament polypropylene. Monofilament polypropylene is not recommended for rope bondage since it is hard and unforgiving. You would best know monofilament as the stuff used to lift crates off of cargo ships! But multifilament is great. When MFP is referred to in this book, we are always referring to multifilament line.

MFP is soft and vibrant in color and its stretch properties are almost identical to nylon, while holding knots slightly better. It is not susceptible to expansion in water, resists damage from many oils and lubricants, and comes pre-dyed in a wide variety of colors. Machine washable and colorfast, MFP can be used in the hot tub without the color fading. I strongly recommend MFP as a bondage rope, especially for

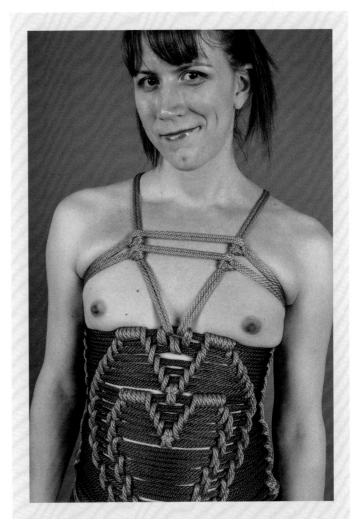

Be as fancy as you want! Erotic macramé is limited only by your creativity.

binding areas that are likely to get exposed to bodily fluids and thus need the rope washed more often.

Ribbon

Though not a form of rope, ribbon of any sort, from vintage lace to present wrapping-ribbon can be used to weave ornate body harnesses, do intricate nonrestraining ties, and coordinate bondage with any outfit. Multi-media decorative bondage can be a delight when combining jute with vintage lace or black MFP with metallic trim.

Sisal

Sisal is a natural-fiber rope made from the leaves of agave plants and has stiff fibers. Though usable on masochists who like splinters or a serious challenge, I do not recommend it for the rest of us.

Silk or Sash Cord

Soft, silky, and perfect for sensuous bondage, sash cord is available in a variety of sizes and colors from fabric supply shops or used clothing stores. It is not in fact silk, but can feel delicious. Actual silk ropes can be fairly expensive and have a fairly low burn speed so fast bondage is not ideal, but if you're seductively binding your lover, it's amazing. Exploring the varieties of exotic materials can be a delight—silk, bamboo, mohair, alpaca, linen, cashmere—so many choices to indulge in.

Webbing

Webbing is a wide, flat material, and comes in cotton, hemp, nylon, polyester and polypropylene. Available in hundreds of colors and patterns, this material is great because it can lay flat along a wider area of the body with fewer wraps around a column. Try it out and explore. Burn speeds vary depending on the type of webbing.

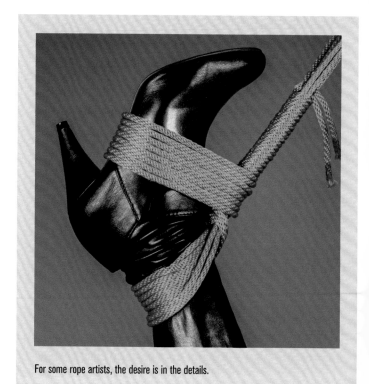

For some rope artists, the desire is in the details.

Length and Width of Rope

There is no perfect length of rope. Your rope needs to be long enough to do whatever job you need done, but you can add on more rope if you run out. If you are just tying a one-column to attach someone to a bed, a 10ft (3+ meter) length piece per wrist is plenty, but each tie is different. I prefer to have a stack of ropes in various sizes available, so I have just the right rope for the job.

To do the ties featured in this book you will need:

- Ball Tie: three 25-30ft (8-10 meter) lengths
- Gyaku Ebi: three 25-30ft (8-10 meter) lengths
- Chair Tie: four 10-25ft (3-8 meter) lengths
- Kani Niwatori: four 25-30ft (8-10 meter) lengths
- Ankle to Wrist: two 10-25ft (3-8 meter) lengths
- Captive Tie: one 25-30ft (8-10 meter) length
- Strap-on Harness: one 25-30ft (8-10 meter) length... and a dildo!

In your toy bag you might include a variety of 10-25 and 25-30ft lengths in multiple materials, along with a pair of EMT shears, blindfold, various sensation toys, a bottle of water, safer sex supplies, a blanket, and whatever else strikes your fancy. All ties shown in this book are done with 6-8mm (1/4" or 3/8") rope.

The trick to choosing the diameter of your rope is knowing what you will be doing with it—if you are mostly tying decorative ties on petite forms, something as small as 4mm can be perfect. If you are doing a moderate amount of wraps on wrists and plan on doing some decorative ties, consider having a mix of 6mm and 8mm in your toy bag. If you want to have your Bottom struggle a lot, or want lines that will look in scale for barrel-chested bodies, consider having a bag full of 8mm and 10mm rope.

Remember—one of the biggest "secrets" in Japanese rope bondage is that you will be folding your rope in half—so 6mm is actually 12mm of coverage per wrap, and 8mm is really 16mm of coverage per wrap. This is why Japanese-style rope bondage tends to use thinner,

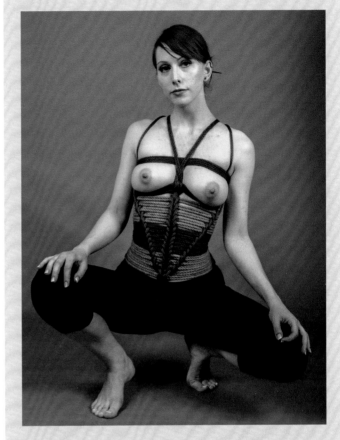

The human body is your canvas—make art that pleases your sense of aesthetics.

longer pieces of rope than its Western single-strand counterpart.

Everyone needs to develop his or her own system. Some artists prefer having a bag made entirely of 10mm 50ft pieces of nylon to reduce the need for adding on extra ropes. Others choose shorter lengths that are less likely to tangle, and are easier to maneuver, adding more rope as needed. Experiment, play around, and take your own path.

Care and Maintenance of Rope

How do you wash your rope? How do you take care of it?

From time to time you will get fluids on your rope—either on crotch ropes, from someone enjoying their bondage quite a lot, or from a spilled beverage. This is when you should consider washing your ropes—and if you play with multiple partners, always wash your rope if it has been exposed to bodily fluids. You may also choose to wash your ropes more often if that is your preference (especially if your ropes get dirty on the ground, or have been in storage for a long time), with an awareness that excessive washing can require replacing ropes more often.

There are two options for washing rope—using a washing machine, and boiling (see page 23). Here is my process for cleaning rope in a washing machine.

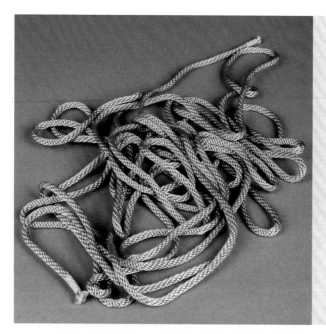

Detangle your rope. This can sometimes be the toughest job of all.

1

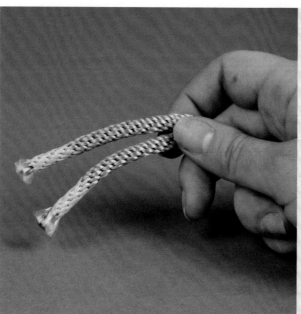

Find the two ends of the rope, thus folding the rope in half.

2

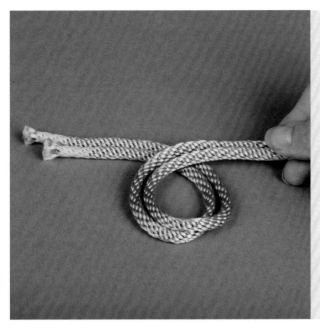

Lay the rope on a flat surface, and make a loop with the loose ends underneath the long folded part of the rope.

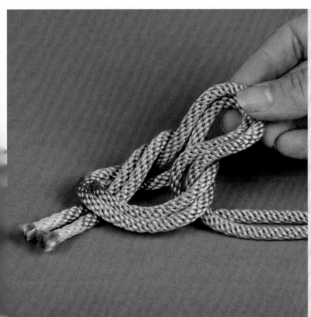

Put your fingers into the loop you have created, and grab some of the line from the long part of the rope. Pull 1-2 inches (3-5 cm) up through the loop.

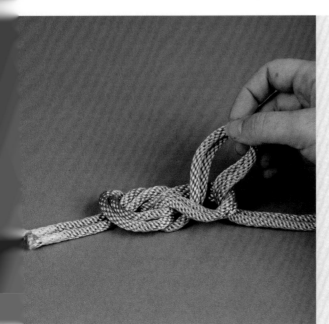

Reach through the newest loop you have just created, grab some of the line from the long part of the rope, and pull it up through the loop.

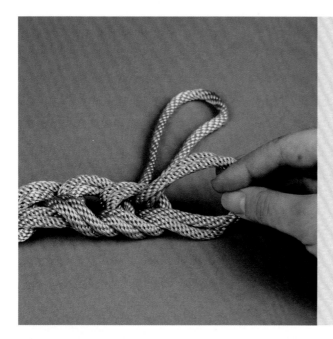

Repeat this process until you have created a long chain of rope. Stop 5-6 inches (12-15 cm) from the folded end (bight) of the rope.

6

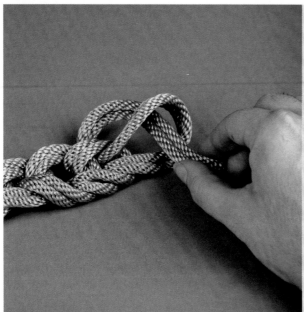

Take the folded end (bight) of the rope and pull it through the last loop you created to keep the chain from unraveling. Pull tight.

7

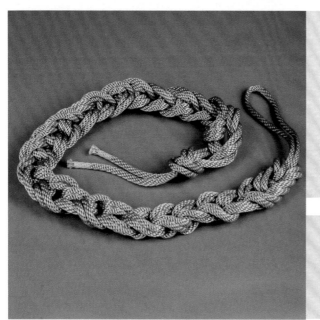

Repeat steps 1-7 with each of the ropes you want to wash.
Take the chain(s) you have made and put them in a lingerie bag (nylon mesh bag used for putting women's lingerie in the washing machine) or a pillowcase (closing with an overhand knot).

8

Throw in washing machine on the medium/warm setting with laundry soap and/or color-safe bleach.

9

Some folks tumble dry their ropes on medium/warm as well. Others dry their rope in the dryer on a setting with no heat. As always, the choice is yours. The other option for washing rope (for rugged natural fibers like hemp and jute) is to boil your ropes. Follow the directions for treating hemp (see page 23) for washing dirty rope.

Gifting dirty ropes to the person whose fluids are on them is also a great option. I recommend that every Bottom have their own crotch rope so that they know that what is between their legs will be clean. If you are unsure if the rope can be cleaned, use a new rope. Your Bottom's health and safety are worth it.

To store your rope, keep it in a cool, dry place away from direct sunlight. You can use a "toy chest," backpack, duffel bag, "toy drawer," or a bin under the bed. If you rarely use your rope, I recommend that you store your ropes loosely coiled/chained so that the ropes do not get bends in them from extended storage.

If you use your ropes regularly, store them in a way that makes them easiest to use. After all, if you are going for style points, it is best for Tops to not have to fumble with, or have to untie knots, mid-scene.

Check your ropes regularly for flaws, damage or debris that may have gotten snagged in them. Ropes get caught on nails, pick up loose material from the floors of dungeons or bedrooms, and simply age with active use. If a rope has a particularly worn point on it, cut it in two—you can make a broken-down 30ft rope into two very usable 15ft ropes this way!

Now that we know how to negotiate our scenes, prepare for a scene, and choose and take care of our rope, let's go tie some folks up!

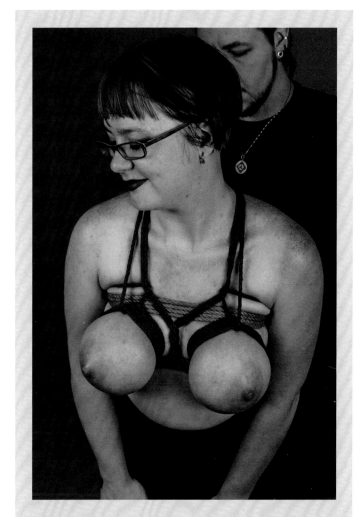

Oh my! This Cupcake Harness (page 56) is a great example of comfortable extreme-looking bondage.

One-Column Ties

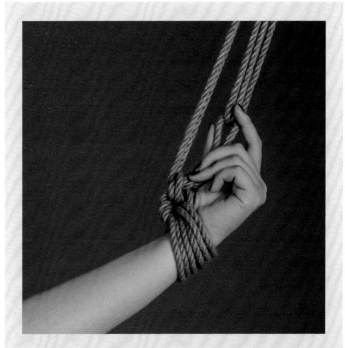

Terminology and Concepts

Before we go through how to tie, here are a few basic terms:

Bight: When a rope is bent double, the point at which the rope folds is called a bight. For the rest of this text, the bight is referring to the bight formed at the middle of the rope when the rope is folded in half.

Cinch: Any rope or action that pulls two pieces of line together. For example, if you have a group of lines running around a pair of wrists, and then you have another line that tightens those wrists towards each other, you have just "cinched" the wrists together.

Column: A column is anything we can wrap rope around: a thigh, an upper arm, a chair leg, etc. Thus, a one-column tie is not a wrist cuff—it is also an ankle cuff, a collar, and a cock-and-ball harness.

Ends: The bit on the rope where the rope stops and the air begins. Ends can be knotted, whipped, dipped, melted, or left to fray.

Line: Slang for a piece of rope, these terms is used interchangeably in the instructional material in this book.

Skein: Also known as a hank or bundle, this term referrs to a single piece of rope when it is coiled up onto itself for easy storage or access. Bundling your rope can reduce the chance of tangling.

Symmetry: To have something be "symmetrical" means it is balanced from side to side. The left side as as many wraps as the right side, for example. Asymmetrical bondage is fun to explore, but for ease of education, most ties in this book are of a symmetrical or near-symmetrical nature.

Tension: The pull or tautness on a rope. When you wrap a rope around a column, it needs to have even tension on every wrap. Having one wrap tight and the next one loose can make your bondage slip, bite into the flesh or cause other difficulties.

A wrist cuff can leave a Bottom feeling erotically exposed, safely held, playfully playing, or straining in their feral power.

Twists: When a rope overlaps itself, gets pulled around itself, or in general does not lay flat. If a rope crosses on top of another rope, it is less comfortable (or can cut off circulation faster) because instead of distributing pressure, the single rope is on the bottom holds the entire pressure for the tie.

Wrap: Any time a line (or in most cases in this text, a pair of lines) is wound around something—whether it is one column, two columns, or anything else—and meets back up with itself, it is considered a wrap.

With these definitions in mind, it is time to get our hands on the rope and start tying!

One-Column Tie

Affectionately known as the boola-boola knot or shibari cuff, this simple tie has a wide variety of applications. It can be tied as a collar and leash, or used to wrap around a thigh to help pull legs back during sexual play.

To have a bit of sexy fun, try putting a wrist cuff on someone and carefully move them around by that cuff to see what poses you can get into. The versatility of just one cuff can fold them over, stretch their body out, or put their hands anywhere the two of you desire.

Another fun game to play with a One-Column Tie is to have a Top bind each of the Bottom's ankles and hand the loose ends to the Bottom. Let the Bottom show you where they would like to take their own body.

The tie here is shown using a 10-15ft (3-5 meter) length of 6mm jute.

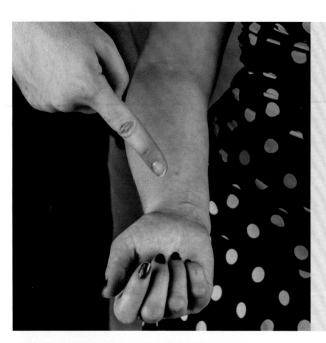

Identify column and find rope

Choose a column. Identify anything you need to avoid, such as joints or the front of a neck.

Find the right piece of rope for what you want to tie—10ft (3+ meters) for binding a wrist to a bed, 25-30ft (8-10 meters) for attaching a thigh up to a headboard. Having rope left over is preferable to having less rope than needed, so err on the side of extravagance when unsure.

1

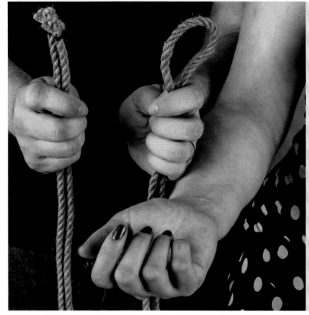

Find the bight

Fold your rope in half and find the bight. Make sure there are no knots in the line and no debris trapped in the rope. Feel the rope for splinters and see what the rope's burn speed is.

2

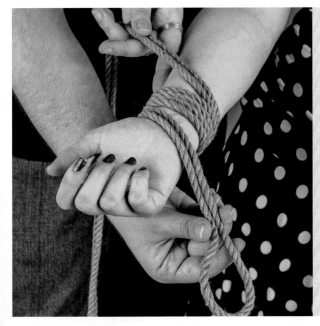

Wrap column

8-12 inches (20-30 cm) from the bight, begin wrapping the folded line around the column. Not too tight mind you; just snug enough to keep the rope from moving. Wrap the column three times to distribute pressure evenly on that column. When wrapped, the rope's lines will resemble the letter "N" or "Z".

3

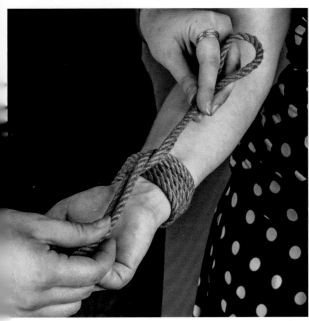

Twist the bight and ends

In a wrist tie, if the bight end was near the hand, it will now be pointing towards the elbow.

4

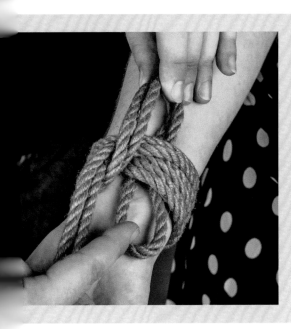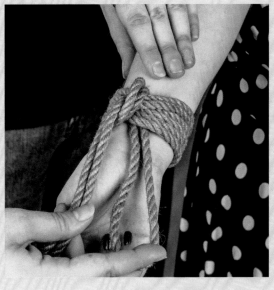

Tuck the bight

Tuck the bight underneath all of the wraps and pull it through.

5

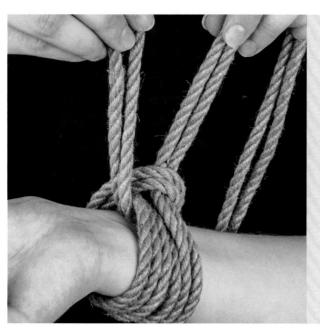

Bring both lines up

This is a great time to see if the wrist ties are as tight as you want. If not, pull the ropes you are holding apart, snug the whole thing down, then bring the lines up once more.

6

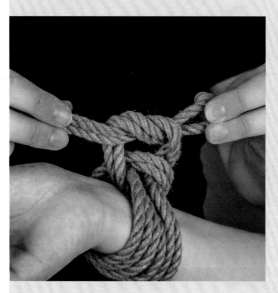 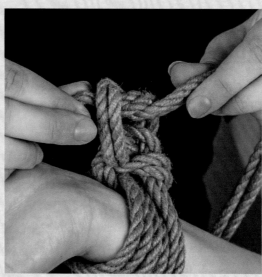

Tie a square knot

Using the bight as one "end" and the loose line as the other "end," tie a square knot (left over right, then right over left). A finished square knot (also known as a reef knot) will resemble the number 8 when viewed from the side. If you are using a slippery line like nylon or MFP, feel free to add an extra overhand knot on top of the square knot to keep it snug.

7

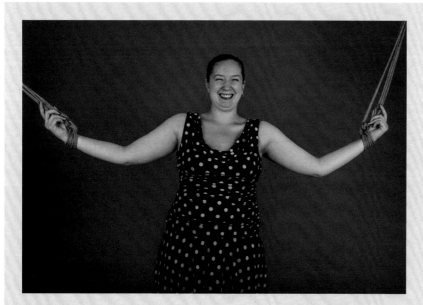

The loop formed by the bight can be used to create a pulley or to tie other lines to, such as running the ends through an overhead point and then back down to the bight loop, and up again. This is perfect for any form of spread-eagle-type ties.

Congratulations! You've just tied your first bit of Japanese-style rope bondage.

Two-Column Ties

This incredibly versatile tie is one of the most used in Japanese-style rope bondage. It goes by many names: rope handcuffs; **Niwatori** (little chicken—when used to tie a wrist to an upper arm); and **Kani** (crab—when used to tie an ankle to a thigh.

Sit down and brainstorm how many columns there are that might be tied. Some will pair up easily by looking at the body symmetrically. Wrist to wrist, ankle to ankle, or even thumb to thumb using Para-Cord. Some require looking at the body asymmetrically, such as binding the wrist to the opposite ankle. Others will go outside the body of one person, attaching one individual to another or tying an ankle to a chair.

As you are practicing new ties, consider doing so outside of the context of a scene or kinky encounter. Grab a piece of rope and try tying your own ankles together. You will gain familiarity with what the rope feels like on someone's skin, as well as how tight you can comfortably pull down on the lines. By having experience before getting into the heat of the moment, you can be more confident and provide a safer experience for your partner.

For some people, the best way to get the information on how to do a tie is based in repetition. By having your hands do the same movements over and over, you gain "muscle memory," where you become able to have your body go on automatic once you start on a technique. Try tying while watching television, hanging out around the house, or when relaxing before bed.

But be forewarned! Don't just practice tying two-column ties as wrist to wrist. Why? Because a mind that has been trained to go on automatic will get confused if you turn it all sideways and try to tie the wrist to the upper arm. If you have done nothing but the wrist to wrist hundreds of times, your body might forget how versatile this technique truly is. Practice—but remember to keep your flexibility as well.

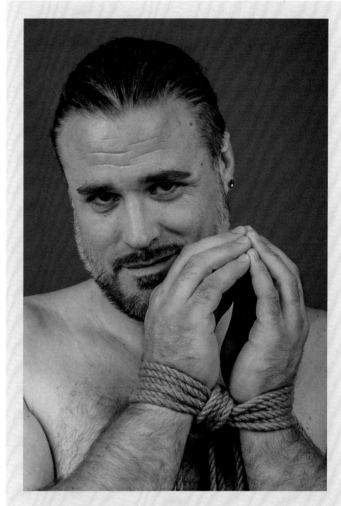

Something as simple as having hands tied can be very sexy.

Basic Two-Column Tie

The Basic Two-Column Tie can be used on a wide variety of columns. The columns need to be parallel to one another, but don't need to be the same width or even be human limbs. The goal of this tie is to lash the columns to one another, maintaining the amount of distance between them. Thus, you can choose two wrists, a wrist and an upper arm, an ankle and a chair leg, as long as the columns have even pressure applied and get locked in place.

When thinking about tying things other than wrists or ankles, consider how snug the space between columns will be. Practice being gentle when learning the Two-Column Tie, so that when you get to binding a thigh to an ankle, you will know how not to pinch or burn more delicate skin. You can always bind more firmly once you get the hang of it.

To tie around the two wrists shown, a 10-15ft (3-5 meter) piece of 6mm jute is shown.

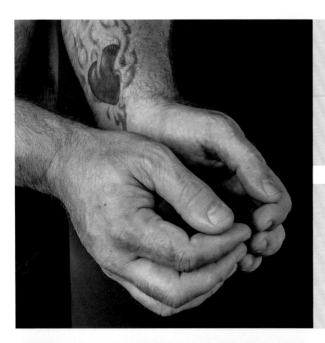

Identify columns

Choose two columns. Identify anything you need to avoid, such as joints or the front of the neck. Make sure to turn the insides of wrists towards each other to protect the arteries, veins and nerves that run close to the surface of the skin.

1

Find your rope

Choose what sort and how much rope you want to use for the tie. If you are tying a pair of thighs together or someone's waist to a tree, you may need a longer piece, 25–30ft (8–10 meters).

2

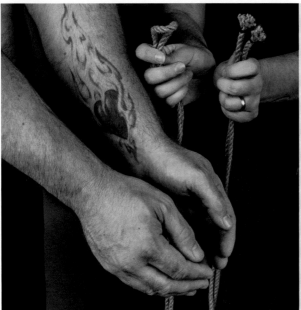

Find the bight

Fold your rope in half and hold the rope by the bight.

3

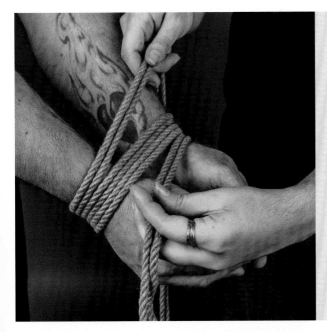

Wrap columns

Wrap the line around both columns with just enough tension to keep the rope from moving. Make sure the columns are not touching one another; they should be anywhere from 1-3 inches (3-7 cm) apart. Wrap the columns three or four times (three wraps are shown in the example) evenly distributing pressure on the columns. When wrapped, the rope will resemble the letter "N" or "Z" with the short/bight end having an 8-12 inch (20-30 cm) tail.

4

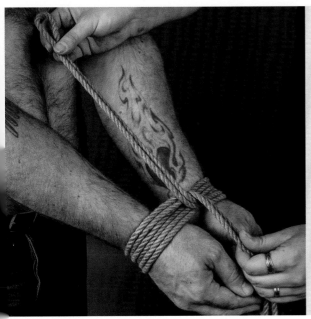

Twist the bight and ends

In a wrist tie, if the bight end was near the hand, it will now be pointing towards the elbow.

5

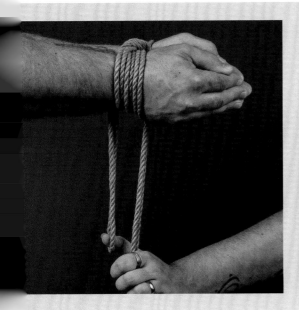
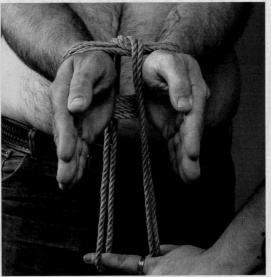

Drop the bight and the ends between the columns

After twisting the bight and ends, bring both the bight and the ends down between the columns.

6

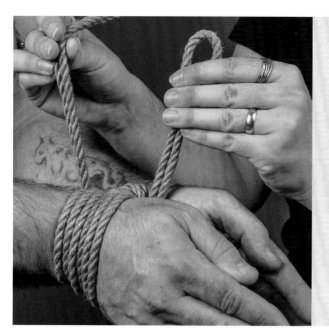

Pull the bight and the ends back up between the columns

If the bight was dropped down near the elbows, pull it back up between the wrists, and vice versa. Make sure the lines lay flat on the opposite side of the wraps from the knot.

7

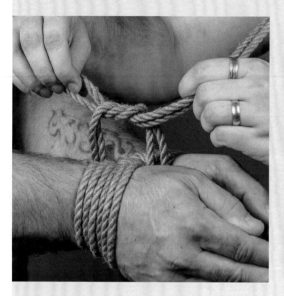
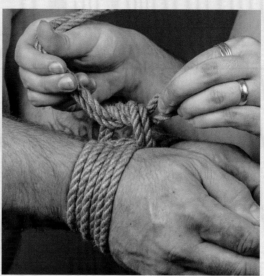

Tie a square knot

Pull the lines between the columns snug, cinching the columns together. Using the bight as one "end" of and the loose ends as the other "end," tie left over right, and then right over left. A finished square knot will resemble the number 8 if viewed from the side. If you are using a slippery line like nylon or MFP, feel free to add a hitch on top of the square knot.

8

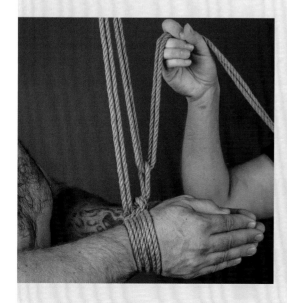
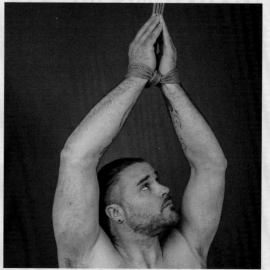

As with a **One-Column Tie**, the loop formed by the bight can be used to create a pulley or to tie other lines to, such as running the ends through an overhead point and then back down to the bight loop, and up again. This is perfect for pulling hands above the head, or tethering to a piece of furniture, as long as the overhead point or furniture can take an appropriate amount of strain for what it is holding.

Variation: Spread Two-Column Tie

There are times when the two columns you want to bind won't quite touch. This variation is great for when an ankle can't reach the thigh, or a pair of wrists don't snug up to one another. The Spread Two-Column Tie is also a great choice for purposefully having space between wrists by creating a spreader-bar out of nothing but rope. Some individuals prefer this modification not out of necessity, but out of aesthetics and flexibility of movement. The ability to move around allows for

Bottoms to assist in taking care of their own health needs while also letting them writhe around seductively. Extra wraps between wrists can lay over breasts framing them, or at the top of the ass framing it nicely. All of those wraps also means more rope marks, which can be a turn-on for some folks.

To tie around the two wrists shown, a 10-15ft (3-5 meter) piece of 6mm jute is shown.

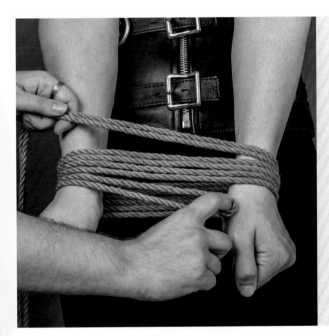

Follow steps 1-4 for **Two-Column Tie** (see page 38)

Start with the columns at 4-10 inches (10-25 cm) apart before you begin wrapping the columns.

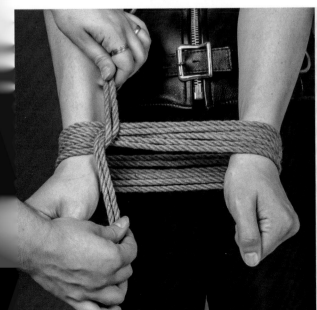

Twist the bight and ends

For a pair of wrists, if the bight end was near the hand, it will now be pointing towards the elbow.

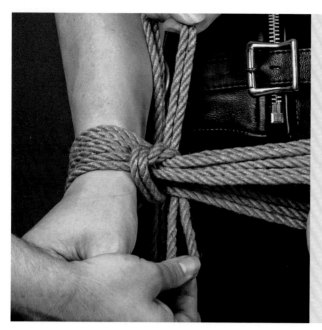

Begin wrapping the bight and ends around the wraps

Wrap the lines in opposing directions, cinching the wraps together as you go. Keep going until you are almost out of rope on the bight end.

6

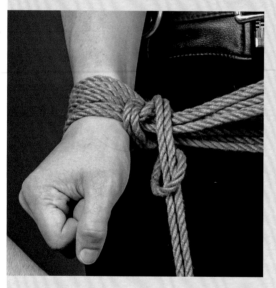

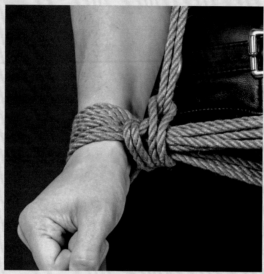

Pull the ends through the bight

Take the ends of the rope and pull them through the bight. Then pull the ends in the direction that pulls the bight tight and keeps tension on the line. If you don't, everything you have tied so far will loosen up. This form of tension on the line is referred to as "reverse tension."

7

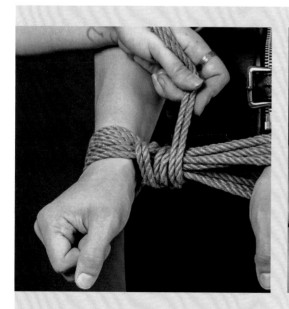

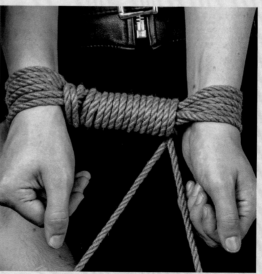

Wrap the line around the wraps

Wrap and wrap and wrap and wrap, keeping everything snug by always pushing back towards the wrist you started from. Keep wrapping until you are snug against the second column. The area next to each wrist should be able to have one finger barely slide in.

8

Split the ends and tuck one through

Split the two ends away from one another. Take one of the ends and tuck it in the gap between the wraps and the second column. Pull it all the way through the gap.

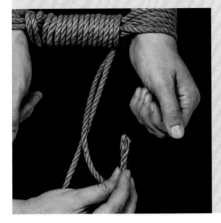
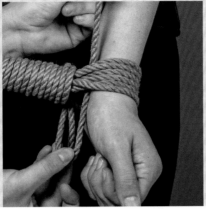
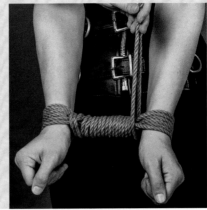

9

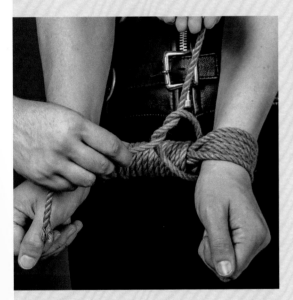
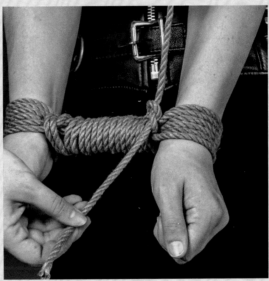

Tie a square knot

Using the ends, tie a square knot. Add an extra hitch if you are using a slippery line. If you are concerned with aesthetics, just tuck the loose ends of the line into open gaps. Have too much rope? Do a second layer of wraps!

10

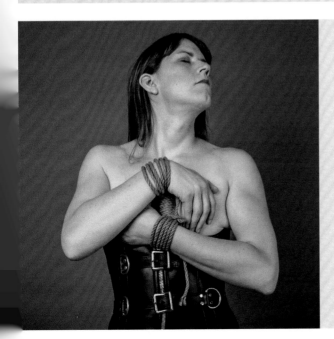

The back side of the wraps should look like this when you're finished. In this version, by struggling she loosened up the wrist wrap lines, but the space between wrists held tight, keeping her bound in the tie.

Shinju (Chest Harnesses)

Shinju translates roughly as "the pearls" and refers to the way that most forms of this chest harness have wraps above and below the breasts or pectorals and then cinch them together. For women with small breasts, this pulls the breasts into tight little balls that resemble pearls.

Chest harnesses, however, can be done on a variety of body types and are great foundations for all sorts of bondage. You can restrict movement of the torso, combine a **Basic Chest Harness** with wrist cuffs (tied using **One-Column Ties**) to pull the hands up behind the back or attach the ankles to the **Box Tie** to form a **Gyaku Ebi** (reverse shrimp tie or Asian hogtie)... the possibilities go on and on.

There is a wide variety of chest harnesses, and in this book we will cover a few different styles:

- Basic Chest Harness
- Clavicle Exposed Chest Harness
- Cupcake Harness (or Big Breast Bondage)
- Box Tie (includes arm and wrist bondage)
- Halter Top Harness
- Small Chest Variation
- Dishevelment

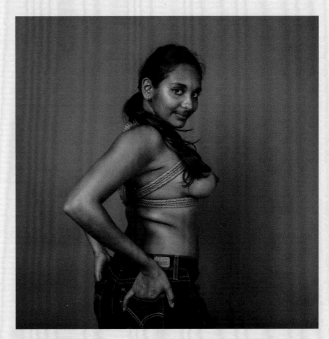

This basic yet elegant chest harness is the beginning template for creating more intricate styles.

When binding the upper body, I have found that the first thing that loses circulation on most people is their hands. Therefore, the **Box Tie** is the only chest harness I have included in this book that begins with the wrists, arms or hands. If having your arms tied back turns you on, I suggest binding the chest and then adding **One-** or **Two-Column Ties** that hold the wrist which attach to the chest harness.

Once you get the hang of the chest harness templates, you will be able to build your own creative applications. The author is right-handed, so the ties are done with that bias. For left-handed individuals, all directions can be reversed left-to-right with no negative effect to structural integrity if so desired.

Basic Chest Harness

The Basic Chest Harness is the framework from which many other chest harnesses are modeled. Some harnesses will have more wraps, cinch in different ways, use different materials or knotting, but they have similar origins. You might be surprised at how simple some sexy images you saw will now be once you can reverse-engineer them with this tie in mind.

Try experimenting once you have played around with this harness. The same tie done in jute will not look or feel the same as tying it in MFP or polyester. See what the tie feels like when the Bottom took a deep breath before being bound as compared to having let all of their breath out. You can learn a lot about each other's desires and bodies by doing such exercises.

This tie was done with a single 30ft (10 meter) length of 6mm jute. However, everyone's body is a different size and shape. For larger frames you may need up to 100ft (30 meters).

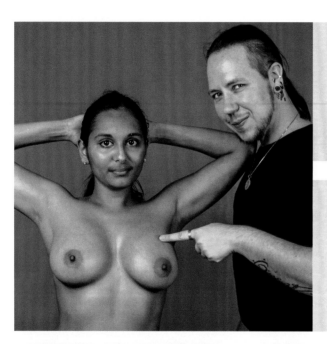

Identify chest

Choose a chest. Identify anything you might need to be aware of, such as breast implants, sensitive nipples, fresh tattoos or piercings, rashes or body hair. Some of these may require minor modifications, such as reducing extreme pressure on breast implants, or pulling rope carefully over body hair.

1

Find your rope

Almost any sort of rope is usable for a chest harness; choose one that you enjoy. If you run out, **adding rope** (see page 53) is always an option. If you have too much, you can add decorative details, clavicle exposure, or wrist restraints with the extra line.

2

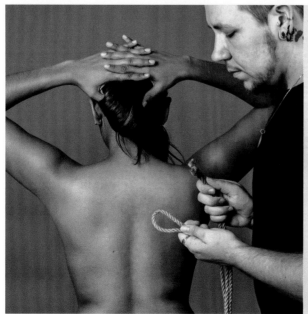

Find the bight

Fold your rope in half. Do whatever menacing or silly thing you like to do as you check the rope for knots, debris, splinters and burn speed. Then, hold the rope by the bight.

3

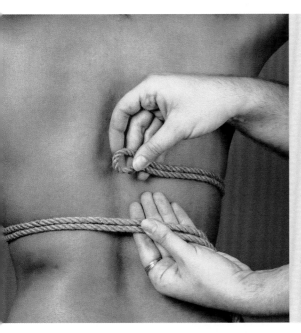

Wrap torso under breasts

With the bight located just to one side of the spine, wrap the folded line around the torso with the ropes just under the breasts. On individuals without breasts, wrap the line a few inches under the nipples, gauging by the line of the pectoral mass.

4

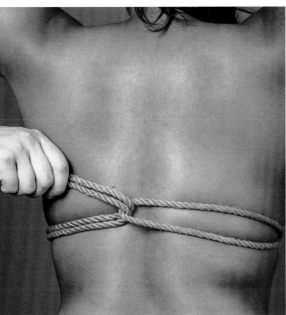

Create lark's head

Pull the ends through the bight, then pull the ends back in the direction that they came from, placing reverse tension on the lines. The lines around the torso should be snug but not restrictive.

5

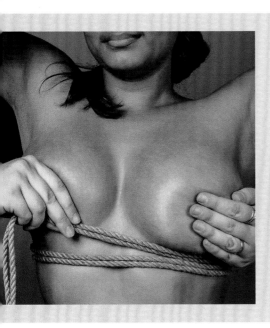
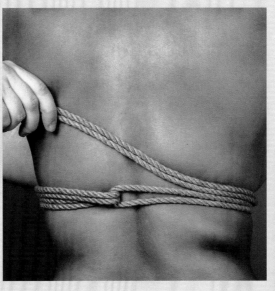

Wrap a second time under breasts

Lay the second set of lines above the first set, just underneath the breasts. You may need to carefully lift the breasts to keep any skin from catching.

6

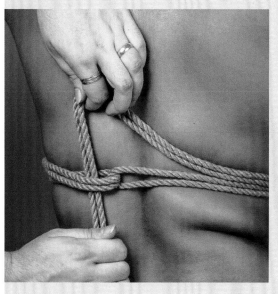 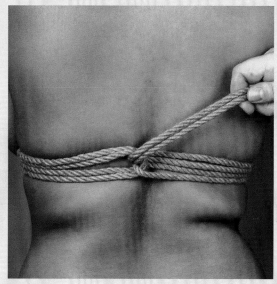

Create second lark's head

When you come back to the first lark's head, you will see that by wrapping a second time, you have created a new loop that rope can be tucked through. Pull the ends through this loop, then pull up and back in the direction the line came from, creating reverse tension.

7

Repeat above breasts

Wrap just above the breast. Tuck ends through the newest loop and pull in the direction the line came from.

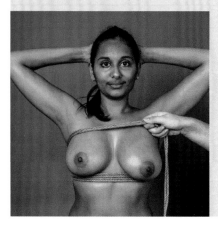 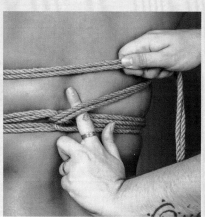 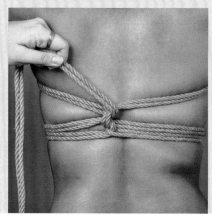

8

Repeat above wraps

Wrap a fourth time, just above the third wrap, and tuck the ends through the newest loop and pull in the direction that line came from.

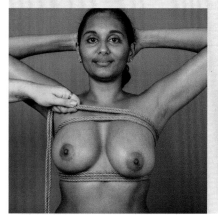 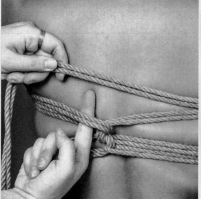 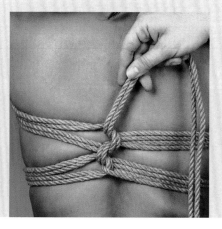

9

Tie off wraps

Hold the rope 2 inches (5 cm) above the chest harness using your right hand and let the ends drop down. Take the loose ends and tuck them up under all of the wraps of the chest harness, pulling the ends through the loop that was just created. Pull the half hitch you have just created tight.

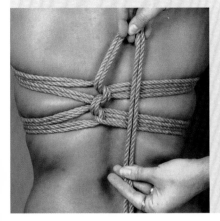 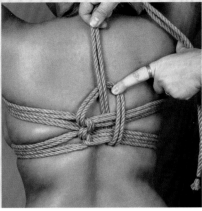 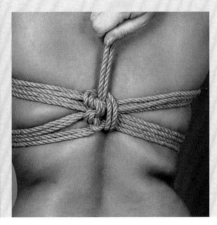

10

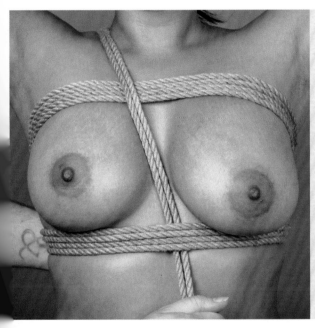

Over shoulder and under lower wraps

Choose a shoulder, any shoulder. In my example, I chose the right shoulder. Tuck the ends underneath the two sets of lower wraps and pull the lines through.

11

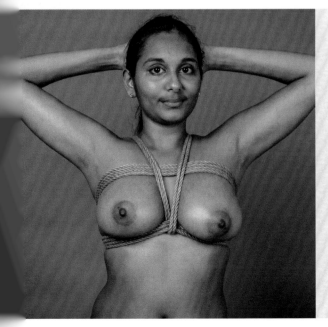

Bring ends up over the other shoulder

In this example, this would be the left shoulder.

12

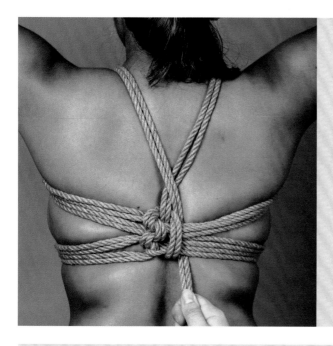

Pull ends under all wraps

Tuck the ends underneath all four sets of wraps and pull through.

13

Tie off shoulder straps

Hold the rope above the chest harness in your right hand and pull the line over with your left hand. Take the loose ends and tuck them underneath both shoulder straps with your left hand, pulling the ends through the loop created with your right hand. Pull the half hitch tight. At this point, your chest harness is finished, but step 15 is included as an idea of what to do with extra rope.

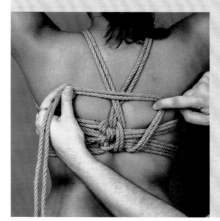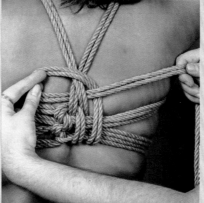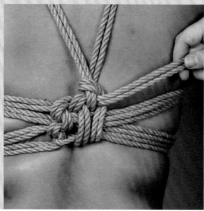

14

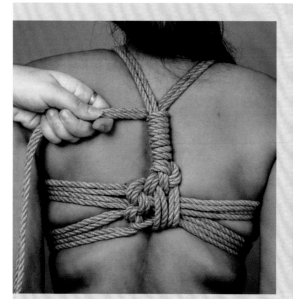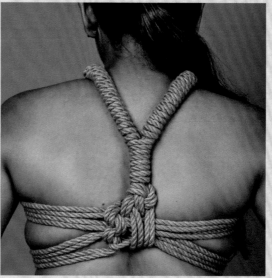

Wrap a whole lot

Take the ends and wrap them around both shoulder straps, then split the lines apart and wrap each line around a different shoulder strap. Other options include wrapping around some of the chest wraps, wrapping around a mixture of chest wraps and shoulder straps or exploring a variety of artistic knotwork.

15

Clavicle Exposed Chest Harness

Having shoulder straps go directly across the collar-bone—the clavicle—can be uncomfortable for some Bottoms. This harness provides a quick and easy fix for this challenge. Once you learn how to do this variation, you can start playing with other ways to move your ropes around.

If this tie takes the shoulder strap and pulls it towards the shoulders, consider what direction you would need to pull from for other modifications to take place. You can pull the upper chest lines up by having the available lines go over the shoulder, catch the upper lines, and then return to the back of the body for example. Play around!

Follow steps 1-14 of the **Basic Chest Harness** (see page 46).

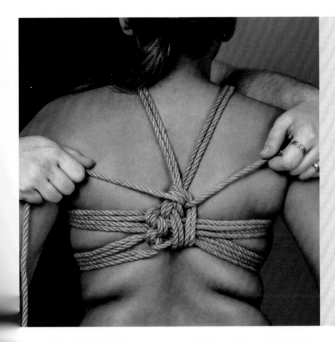

Split the lines

Once the lines from the shoulder straps are tied off with a half hitch, have one line run to the left and one to the right, above the four sets of wraps that went around the torso.

15

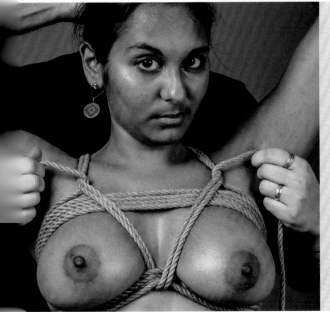

Pull ends underneath shoulder straps

Having gone underneath the left armpit, pull the left rope ends underneath the left shoulder strap, then pull it back in the direction it came from. The goal is to pull the shoulder strap off of the collarbone and reduce tension on the upper front of the chest. Repeat on the right side.

16

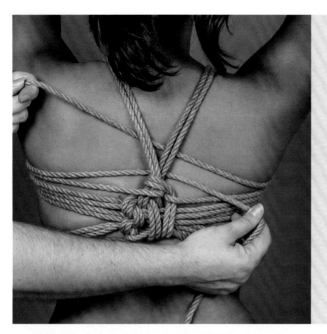

Return to back and go under shoulder straps

Tuck the end of the left line under both shoulder straps, passing over to the right side. Repeat with the other line. Tension on both ropes should be even, with symmetrical clavicle pulling on the front of chest.

17

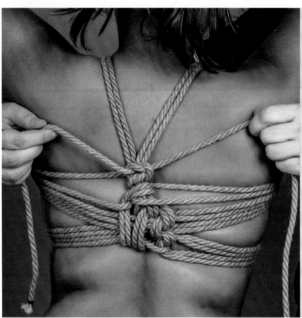

Tie a square knot

Take each line and use them to tie a square knot (see page 36).

18

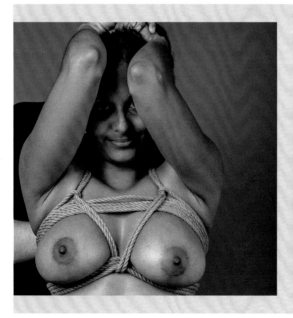

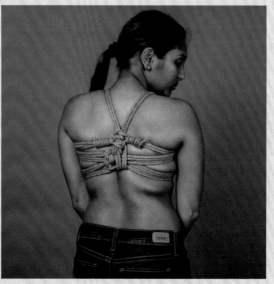

Wrap a whole lot

Take the ends and wrap them around the lines from the clavicle pull. Other options include wrapping around the chest wraps, around a mixture of chest wraps and shoulder straps, going around shoulder straps, or using knotwork that expresses your artistic vision.

19

Adding Rope Option 1:
Overhand with Lark's Head

We've run out of rope! What are we supposed to do?

No fear! We can always add on extra rope.

Running out of rope is a very common occurrence, and there is nothing wrong with it happening from time to time. If you think you need three pieces of rope for a scene, have four or five with you. It allows for when you happen to mismeasure, when a rope tangles, or if you come up with a new idea.

Taking a moment to add on new ropes is also a great chance to pause and touch your partner, reminding them that you know there is a person inside all of that rope. Sometimes Tops can get so fixated on getting the bondage "right." These natural pauses allow for an opportunity to reconnect.

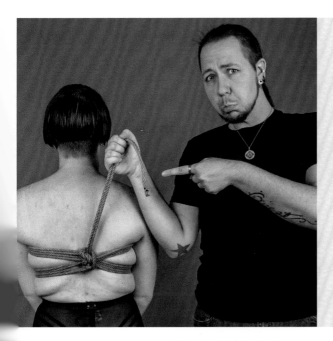

Oh no! We've run out of rope!

Well... let's start with that rope that we're holding already, shall we?

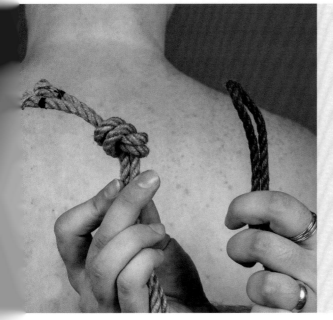

Find the bight on the second rope

Tie a single overhand knot near the ends of the lines you are already working with. If the second rope you are adding is significantly larger in diameter, tie two overhand knots on top of one another.

Find a second rope, and fold that rope in half.

1

Make a lark's head in second rope

Place your thumb and index finger inside the bight of the second rope. Spread your thumb and index finger apart. Rotate your hand so that your fingers are now facing down and the doubled line is between your thumb and index finger. Bring your thumb and index finger together, sliding both loops onto your index finger and middle finger. This creates the lark's head.

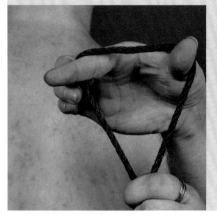
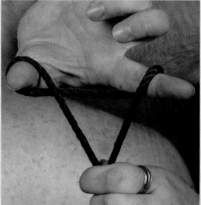
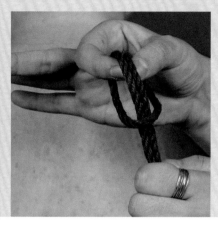

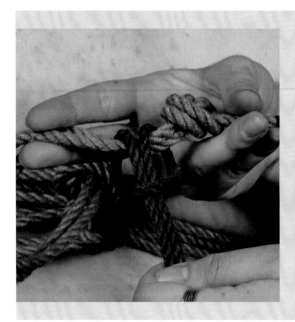
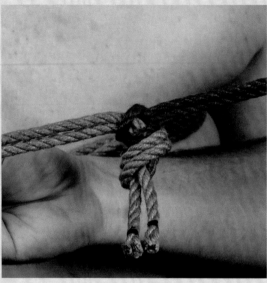

Slide lark's head over overhand knot

Grab the overhand knot between your index finger and middle finger and slide the lark's head over the overhand knot. Tighten the lark's head down. You now have a longer rope!

Adding Rope Option 2:
Lark's Head to Main Body

There are times when continuing off of the rope you have been working with is not desired. Perhaps the lines you were working with ended up being tied to one another. Maybe you want to pick up tying somewhere in a different part of the bondage, beginning at the front of the tie rather than on the back for example (see page 92 for an example).

You might also want to use this specific technique because it lays very flat across the body, and can be tied around one segment of rope, or many. Try playing with both of these techniques for adding rope to see which one works best for you in which situations. Varieties of technique allow for more combinations as you evolve in your rope knowledge.

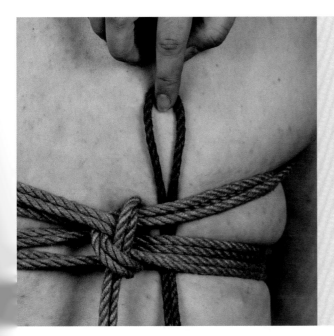

Slide bight under wraps

Choose a second rope and hold the rope by the bight. Slide this folded line under all of the chest wraps, or just a few—whatever works best for the given situation.

1

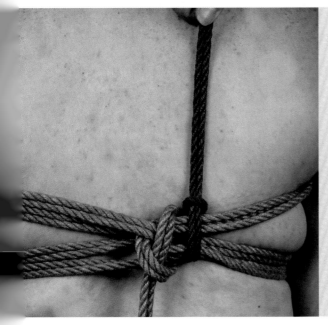

Pull ends through bight

By pulling the ends through the bight and snugging down, you create a lark's head. You are now free to keep going.

2

Cupcake Harness

For individuals with a breast size of C-cup or larger, carefully and sensually wrapping each breast can dramatically focus attention to this part of the body. This harness shows a way to secure those breast wraps so that they do not slip around by attaching them at multiple points to a modified **Basic Chest Harness.**

Though the tie may look visually intense, the tie should not be painful without that being a consciously added part of the scene. If you wrap tightly around

the breasts, the skin will begin discoloring. It is possible to pop capillaries which creates little red dots on the skin's surface, especially if you do any impact play (slapping, caning) with the bound breast. Additional care should be taken when wrapping breasts on individuals with breast implants.

An additional 30ft (10 meter) piece of rope was added to the **Basic Chest Harness** to convert that tie into this more detailed form.

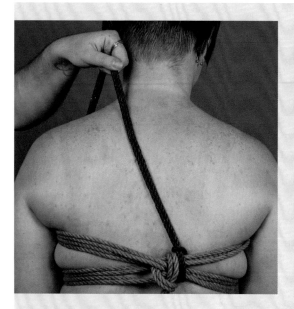 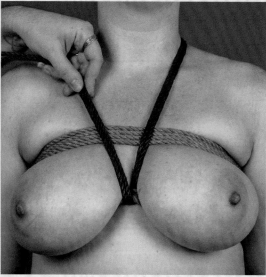

Follow steps
1-10 of the **Basic Chest Harness** (see page 46).

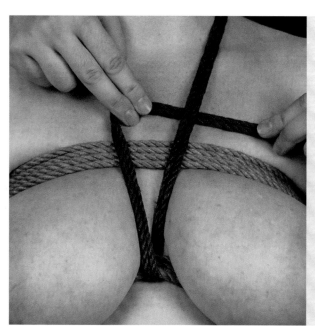

Pull ends underneath shoulder strap

Make sure your Bottom is not looking at the chest harness when you do this or else you risk hitting her in the eye if the ends come through at a high speed.

11

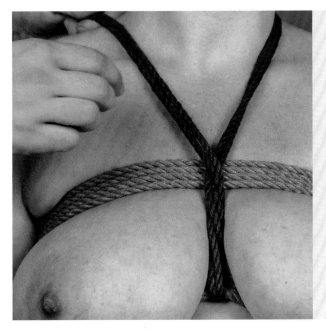

Snug and drop ends over other shoulder

By adding that extra tuck of rope, you have created a decorative twist in the front of the chest harness. Snug the twist down and drop the ends over the other shoulder.

12

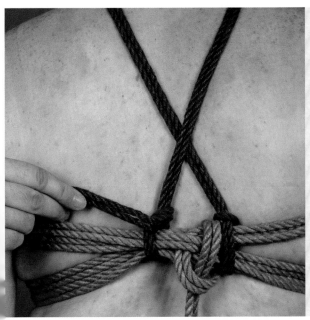

Tie off shoulder straps

Use an overhand knot to tie off around the torso wraps. Tying off around both shoulder straps as shown in **step 14** of the **Basic Chest Harness** (see page 50) is also a valid option.

13

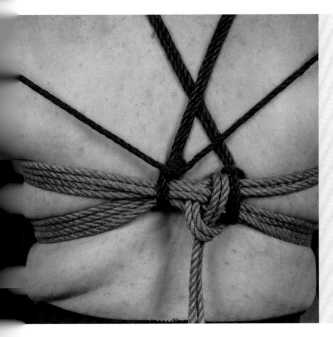

Split the lines

Once the lines from the shoulder straps are tied off, have one run to the left and one to the right, above the four sets of wraps that went around the torso, just as you did in the **Clavicle Exposed Chest Harness** (see page 51).

14

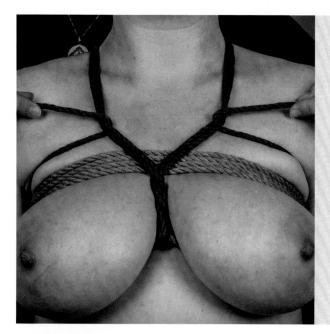

Pull ends underneath shoulder straps

Pull the left side's end underneath the left shoulder strap, then create reverse tension. Our goal is to anchor the rope above the breasts so we can bind each breast independently. Repeat on the right side.

15

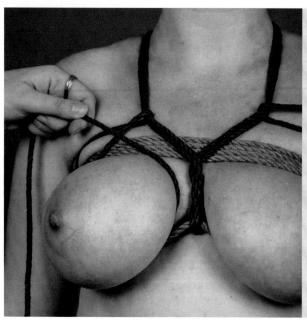

Wrap right breast

Hold her right breast in your right hand while slowly wrapping the line around the breast towards the outside of the body. Get the rope as snug to the torso as possible when passing under the breast. Ask your Bottom how snug you can wrap, as everyone has different thresholds and desires for this sort of bondage.

16

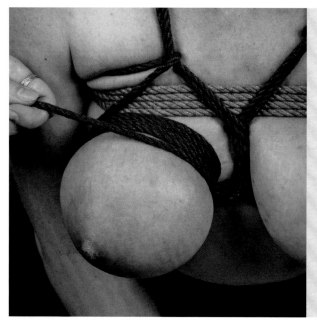

Continue wrapping right breast

Make sure your lines lay right up against one another as you wrap, with no gaps between lines. Stop wrapping when you are either near the end of your line, you run out of breast to wrap, or you are happy with how the harness looks.

17

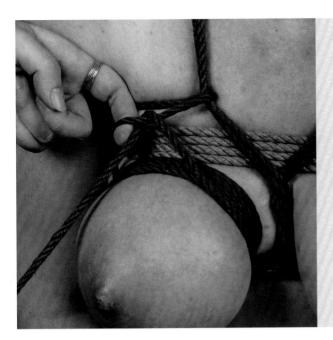

Tuck end underneath clavicle pull

Pull the rope under the lower clavicle pull line that was laid in **step 15**.

18

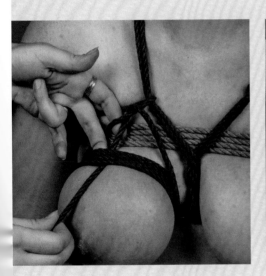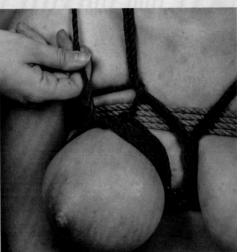

Tuck line underneath all the breast wraps

Pulling from next to the chest towards the nipple on the right breast, gently slide the end underneath all the breast wraps. If the wraps are very tight, you may have to tuck the line under one wrap at a time. Make sure not to pull through too fast, lest you cause abrasion.

19

Bind the left breast

Repeat steps 16-19 on the left breast, holding the breast in your left hand and wrapping around the breast in the opposite direction that you did the first breast. Wrap the same number of times as you did on the right breast, then tuck the end underneath the clavicle pull and all of the breast wraps.

20

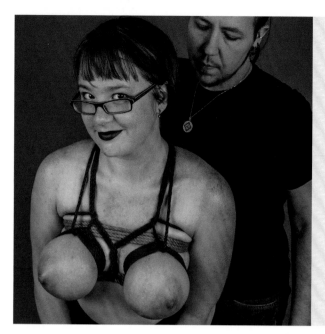

Create shoulder straps

Run the lines from the breast bondage up over each shoulder, lifting the breasts as you do so. This will add snugness to the bondage, and position each breast in the "cupcake" position.

21

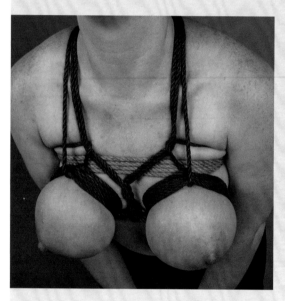

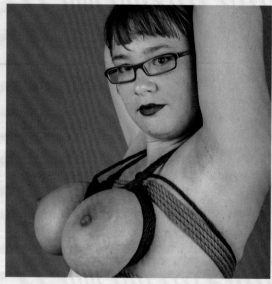

Tie off

Take each line and use them to tie a square knot on the back side. The finished product should appear similar to this on the front and side.

22

Box Tie

Sometimes referred to as a "simplified takate kote," the Box Tie takes its name from the box-shaped arm position the Bottom holds when bound. This version of the Box Tie allows for a fairly swift release of the hands if circulation is lost, without the entire chest harness having to be undone.

The Bottom will need to be able to have their inner wrists (or better yet, their inner forearms) overlap to create the Box Tie. If the Bottom is able to have their hands reach the opposite elbow, they should not "lock" their thumbs into their opposite "elbow-pit." Not every person can hold this specific pose, but the same stylistic effect can be achieved by tying a **Basic Chest Harness** and then using a **One-Column** Tie to pull each wrist upward.

This tie was done with two 30ft (10 meter) lengths of 6mm jute. For larger frames you may need up to 120ft (35 meters).

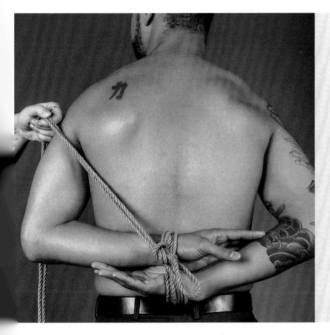

Tie wrists as single one-column tie

Tie a **One-Column Tie** (see page 34) around both wrists. The cuff shown here should be loose enough to give the Bottom space to wiggle around if they get uncomfortable. Doing so allows for some reduction of circulation and nerve concerns.

1

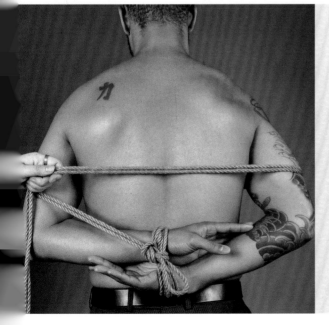

Wrap torso under breasts and over arms

Wrap the doubled line around the torso and upper arms with the ropes just under the breasts or pectoral mass.

2

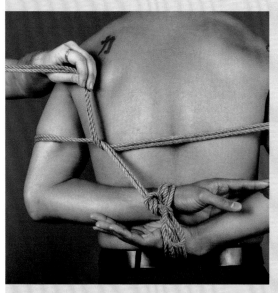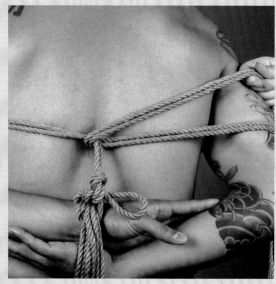

Make a lark's head

Tuck the ends underneath the line that comes up from the wrist, then pull the ends back in the direction that they came from. Continue to pull until the line from the wrist creates a straight line up the spine to create the "box" shape.

3

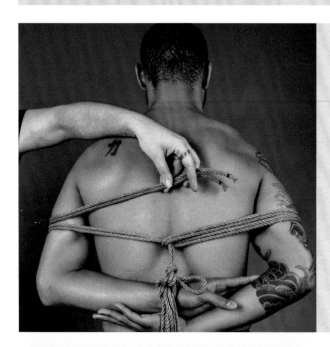

Wrap a second time under breasts

Lay the second set of lines above the first set, just underneath the breasts. Lift the breasts to keep any skin from catching if needed.

4

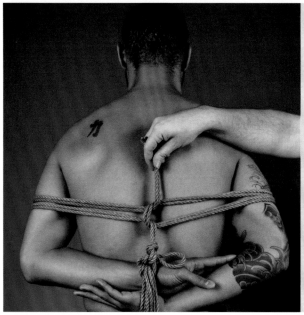

Create second lark's head

When you come back to the first lark's head, you will see that by wrapping a second time, you have created a new loop that rope can be tucked through. Pull the ends through this loop, then pull up and back in the direction the line came from, creating reverse tension. These lower two wraps should be near the halfway point on the upper arm, reducing the chance of nerve pressure.

5

Repeat steps 4 and 5 twice above breast

Add rope (see page 53) if needed, then wrap just above the breast. Tuck ends through the newest loop and pull in the direction the line came from. Wrap a fourth time, just above the third wrap, and tuck the ends through the newest loop and pull in the direction the line came from. The fourth wrap should line up with or near the armpit in front.

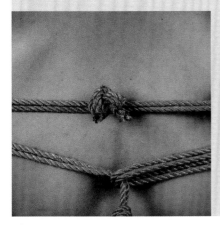
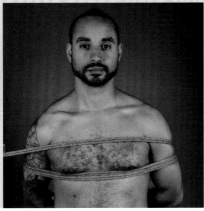
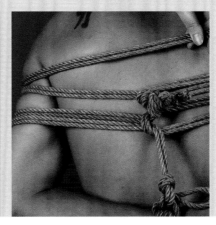

6

Tie off wraps

Tie a half hitch around all four sets of chest ropes.

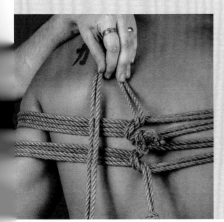
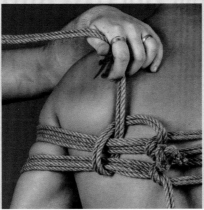
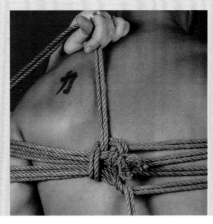

7

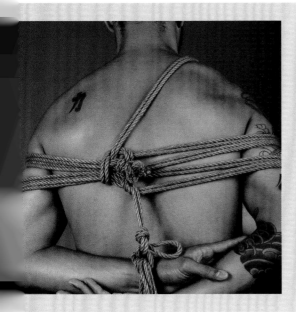
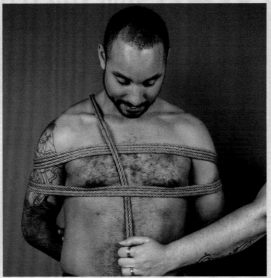

Over shoulder and under lower wraps

Choose a shoulder, any shoulder. In my example, I chose the right shoulder. Tuck the ends underneath the two sets of lower wraps and pull the lines through.

8

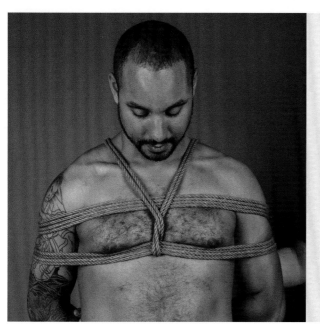

Snug and drop ends over other shoulder

Create a decorative twist in the front of the chest harness by bringing the rope up on the side of the body that you came from (in this case, the right side of the body) before tucking it under the rope you just laid. Having done so, drop the ends over the other shoulder.

9

Tie off shoulder straps.

Tuck the ends underneath all four sets of wraps and pull through. Add additional rope as needed at any point during this bondage, unless the knot will be placed on a tender part of the body such as between the torso and underarm. Pull the line upwards, and tie a half hitch around both sets of shoulder straps. Pull tight.

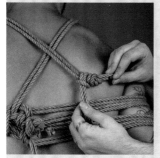
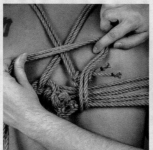
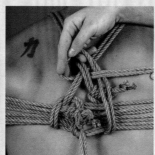
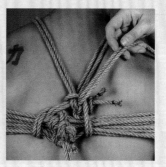

10

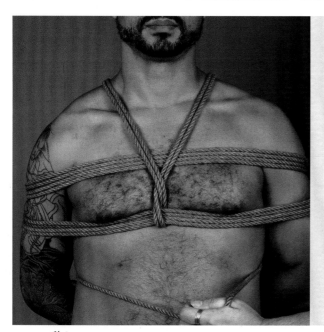

Split and run line between arm and torso

Take one strand run it to the left while running the other and to the right, just below the four sets of wraps that went around the torso. Use the gap at the "elbow-pit" to have less friction as you pull through.

11

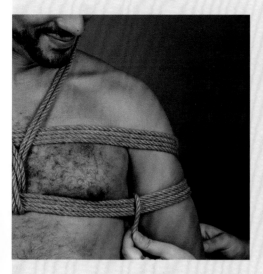
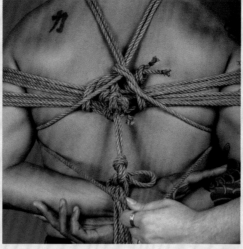

Tuck line between upper and lower torso wraps

Pull the end of the line up into the space between the doubled sets of torso wraps. Pull the line back down, creating pressure on the lower sets of torso wraps as you pass the line back through the elbow pit. If working with someone that might slip the upper sets of torso wraps off over their shoulders, the line can be pulled under both sets of doubled wraps.

12

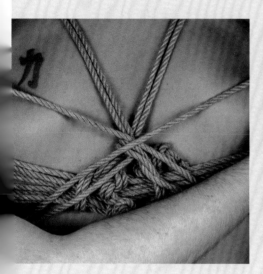
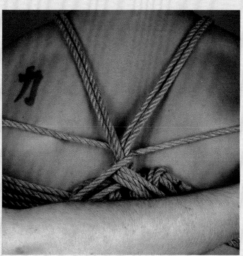

Tuck ends underneath shoulder straps

Tuck the line that ran underneath the left arm under the shoulder straps from left to right. Tuck the line that ran underneath the right arm under the shoulder straps from right to left.

13

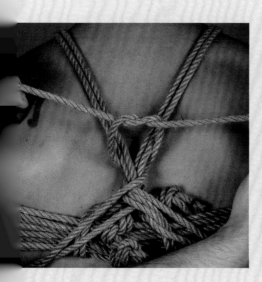
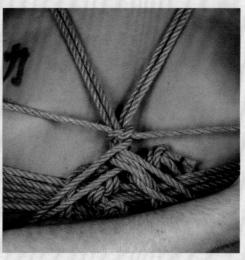

Tie a square knot

Tie a square knot around the shoulder straps. Feel free to add an extra hitch on top of the square knot if you're using a slippery line.

14

Catch the One-Column loop

When you tied the **One-Column Tie** in **step 1**, a small loop was left exposed. Run your extra rope down through the loop before bringing the line back up. Unless this loop is caught and brought up, the wraps around the torso could tighten if the Bottom's hands drop.

15

Wrap a whole lot

In this example, I wrapped the ends around the shoulder straps before tying off with a square knot and tucking the ends away. The finished product should appear similar to this on the back, side, and front.

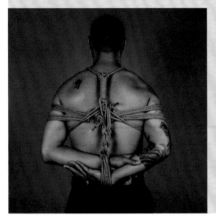
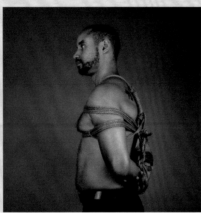
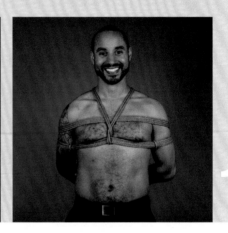

16

But what should I do if their hands fall asleep?

If your Bottom reports numbness in their hands, you can release the hands without undoing the harness. Untie anything that attaches the shoulder or torso lines to the wrist tie, untie the wrist cuffs and let the hands go—the rest of the bondage can stay in place. If you want to put your Bottom back in the same pose after their circulation returns, just re-tie the wrist cuff—voilà!—you're back in business.

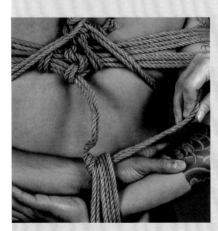
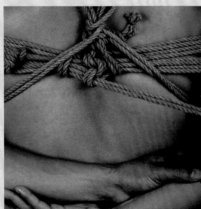
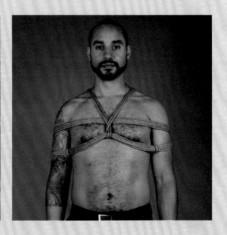

Sometimes the original position isn't an option any more. Consider tying their hands in front instead, using a **Two-Column Tie** in front of their belly, attaching the wrists to one another. You can also attach their wrists to their upper thigh using a **Two-Column Tie** on each side for another variation. Have fun with it, and see what works for their body and your desires alike.

Halter Top Harness

here are times when having all of your knots in front [is] preferred. Your partner might have an amazing tattoo [y]ou want to "frame" across their shoulders. Your flogger [is] in the cards for tonight's scene, and you don't want [th]e leather falls hitting on top of the ties. Perhaps your [p]artner will be lying on their back, and they tend to [n]otice those bumps behind them.

[Alt]hough it is possible to use pillows to prop up around [kn]ots and make rope bondage more comfortable all

around, this fashion-forward and aesthetically pleasing tie offers another choice. Think of it as your own erotic bikini top! Use this concept as the jumping off point for crafting chest harnesses outside of the classic model. Make your own fashion, create your own designs, and have fun!

This tie was done with a single 30ft (10 meter) length of 6mm MFP rope.

Wrap torso four times

Follow a similar pattern from **steps 1-9** from the **Basic Chest Harness** (see page 46), except all lark's heads will be in the center of the chest instead of the middle of the back, starting with the wraps above the breasts rather than under the breasts. By doing so, you start at the top, and work your way down.

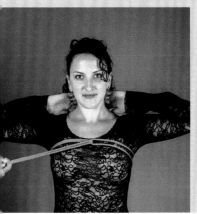
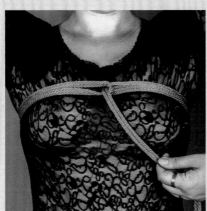
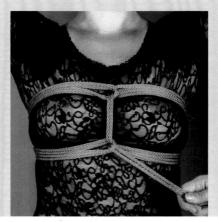

Tie off wraps

Hold the rope 2 inches (5 cm) below the lower chest wraps in your left hand.
Tie a half hitch around the ropes that run under the breasts. Pull tight.

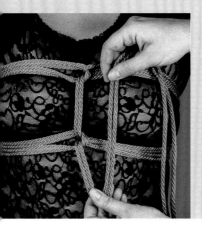
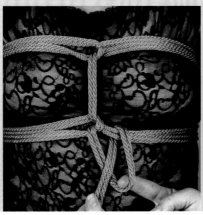
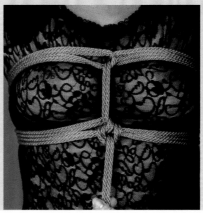

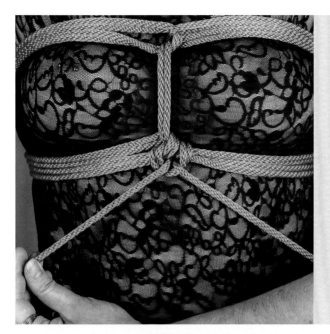

Split the lines

Once the lines from the torso wraps are tied off, have one run to the left and one to the right, just below the two sets of wraps that went around the torso below the breasts.

3

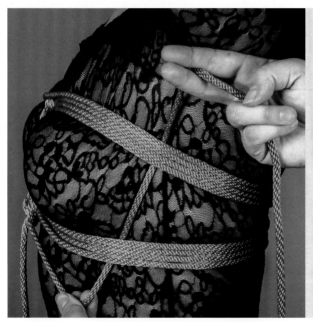

Tuck ends underneath torso wraps on sides

From bottom to top, tuck the end underneath the sides of the torso wraps and pull snug. This will create an "underwire" effect on individuals with breasts. If there is not enough breast tissue present to create this effect, the line will end up creating a diagonal stripe across the chest, crossing near the nipple.

4

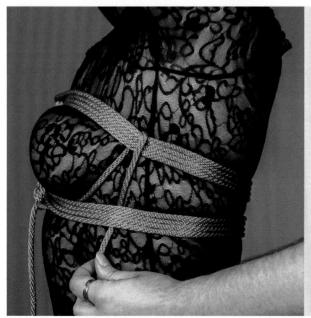

Tuck underneath lower torso wraps

From top to bottom, tuck the end underneath the lower torso wraps and pull snug.

5

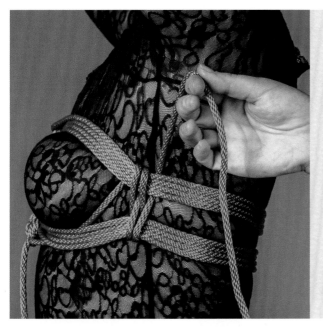

Tuck underneath upper torso wraps and repeat

From bottom to top, tuck underneath the upper torso wraps and pull snug. **Repeat steps 5 and 6** once more to create a band of wraps on the side of the chest. With the left side completed, repeat the underwire and side wraps on the right side.

6

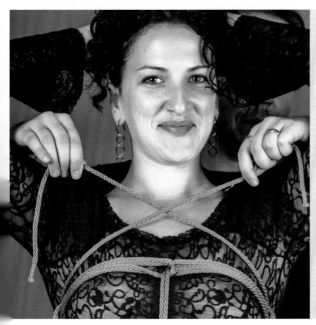

Cross lines over chest

Run the line from the right side of the torso over the left shoulder, and the left side of the torso over the right shoulder.

7

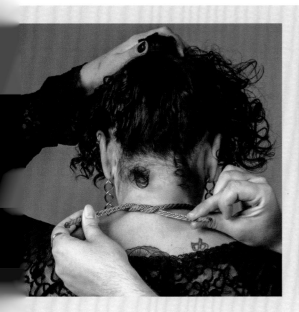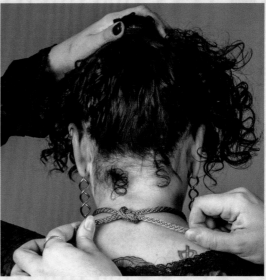

Tie square knot behind neck

Take each line and use them together to tie a square knot directly behind the neck.

8

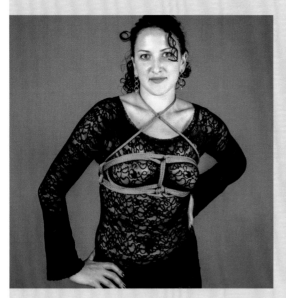
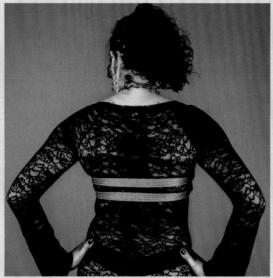

The finished product should appear similar to this on the front and back.

Small Chest Variation

The goal on this tie is to create wide decorative elements that fill the open space on the smaller chested individual and yet not have any bulky knots that would detract the eye from the breasts themselves.

In this variation, I began with only one wrap above and below the breasts. I split the lines before going over the shoulders, then brought the lines back together to go under and then over the lower torso wraps. The lines crossed over each other before changing directions, the formerly left line becoming the new right shoulder strap, and vice versa. Returning to the back, they were tied off, and then I created a variation of the clavicle pull. The clavicle line came up to one of the shoulder straps, twisted around it, then became a third shoulder strap. I returned both lines over the shoulders they came from and tied them off in the back.

Finding your own ways to creatively modify these ties to the body of your partner will let them know that you are thinking about them when you are tying. Thus, whether you choose to replicate ties in this book identically, or modify the chest harnesses, it is about making rope yours.

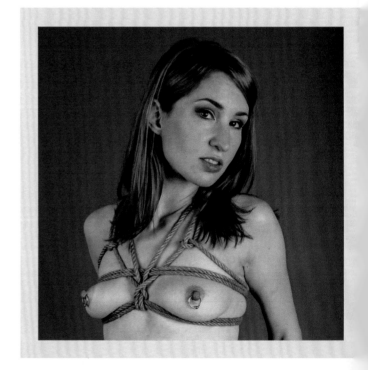

Dishevelment

One of the themes in Japanese-style rope bondage is dishevelment and distress. In pornography, you will often see images of women with kimonos pulled open, pantyhose partially pulled down on one side, or hair tousled and out of place. Polka-dotted dish rags get used as gags or blindfolds, enema rigs are hanging nearby, and looks of anguish and shame are shown for a titillating effect.

An option to create an air of dishevelment begins with a perfectly pristine woman (or man). Bind her, then expose her flesh after she is tied, leaving her hair pulled out of place and her body on display "against" her wishes. Remember, this is about desire, fun, and role-play, not about actually taking anyone against their will... but the effect can be delicious.

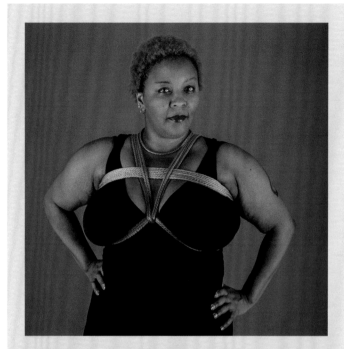

Have your Bottom wear a robe, button-down shirt, a loose shirt or dress... or perhaps an item of clothing that you can destroy. In this case, I chose to have my Bottom wear a loose dress. I tied a variation on a **Basic Chest Harness** (see page 46) over her clothed torso. Once she was tied, I then began to pull her top down while whispering in her ear what I longed to do to her. I pulled the fabric away to expose each breast in turn.

Her reaction was more playful, but for Bottoms who are new to rope, or who long to feel consensually degraded, it can be embarrassing, humbling, or arousing. Remember that classical Shibari draws its erotic degradation from the iconography of its own culture. Look around at your own culture for inspiration. Look at what is in your own kitchen, bathroom and garage for ideas!

All right. Now that we have these delightful chest harnesses to choose from, let's move on to some fun combinations, shall we?

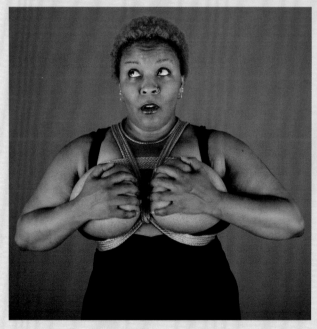

Combinations

Now that you know how to do one-column ties, two-column ties and a variety of chest harnesses, there is a wide variety of possible combinations you can try. In the following pages, you will see ideas for mixing and matching these elements into these combinations:

- Gyaku Ebi (Reverse Shrimp—Asian Style Hogtie)
- Ebi or Kuri (Shrimp or Ball Tie)
- Chair Tie
- Kani (Crab)
- Niwatori (Little Chicken)
- Ankle to Wrist Tie
- Captive Tie (binding both hands at the back of the head)

As you look at bondage erotica and pornography online, you will see that much of what is shown uses a variety of the base ingredients that you have learned so far. Feel free to be inspired by the classic combinations offered in this chapter, as well as what you see others producing.

Each time you learn a new tie, you will be adding a new ingredient to your palette of possibilities. What you cook up is up to you. Collaborate with your partner and see what ideas they have as well. So often we expect Tops to have all of the ideas for scenes. Bottoms usually have beautiful, sensual, or wicked concepts brewing as well. Curling up and whispering fantasies, or setting aside "practice time" to try out new rope concepts can help transfer the material from one partner to the other.

It doesn't have to be perfect every time you experiment. Sometimes our most beloved ideas come to us when we are trying out something that didn't quite work. Have fun. Connect with your lover. Play around. See what you come up with as you find your own style.

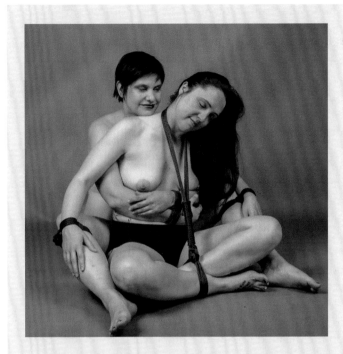

Combinations can be used to bind more than one person at a time.

Gyaku Ebi (Reverse Shrimp)

The Gyaku Ebi, also known as the Reverse Shrimp Tie or Asian Style Hogtie, is an incredibly versatile form of bondage. Unlike the "Western" hogtie—which binds the wrists together, then attaches the ankles to the bound wrists—the pull of the ankles does not risk the chance of dislocating your Bottom's wrists. All of the tension lies across the chest harness, a much wider area for the distribution of pressure.

When you tie a Gyaku Ebi, you can choose to have the hands tied first (as in the **Box Tie** shown here) or bound after the chest harness is tied. The second option alleviates stress on the arms that may be caused by the pull of the legs on the chest harness. If someone has a larger frame or cleavage, consider using pillows to prop up the other parts of them to help them breathe with more ease.

In these images, the person on his knees had to focus on his balance to stay upright. Gyaku Ebi is intended predominantly for an individual on his belly or sides, and the Bottom should not be expected to stay upright for extended periods. As with all bondage, no one in a tie like this (upright or on the belly) should be left alone.

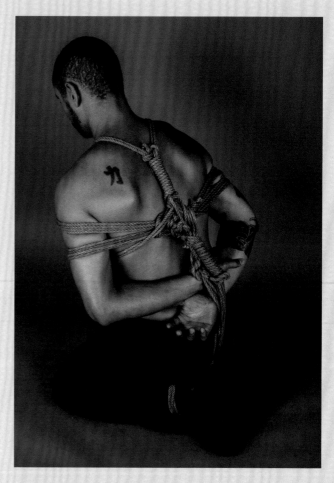

· Upright Gyaku Ebi

Bind upper body

Restrain the upper body and hands. The **Box Tie** (see page 61) is shown here.

1

Tie the ankles together

The **One-Column Tie** (see page 34) is a good option, though the **Two-Column Tie** (see page 38) is also a valid choice. Sexual play can be explored by having each ankle tied separately to the chest harness.

2

Attach ankles to chest harness

Run the ends from the ankle tie underneath all of the torso wraps.

3

Create pulley system

Run the ends from the chest harness back down to the loop from the **One-Column Tie**. Using the bight, create a pulley system that helps move the rope more quickly and easily. Every Bottom has a different amount of flexibility and tension they can endure. Check in with them as you cinch down to make sure you do not hurt their knees or chest, or impair their ability to breathe.

4

Tie off

Use an overhand or square knot to tether the cinched ropes in place.

5

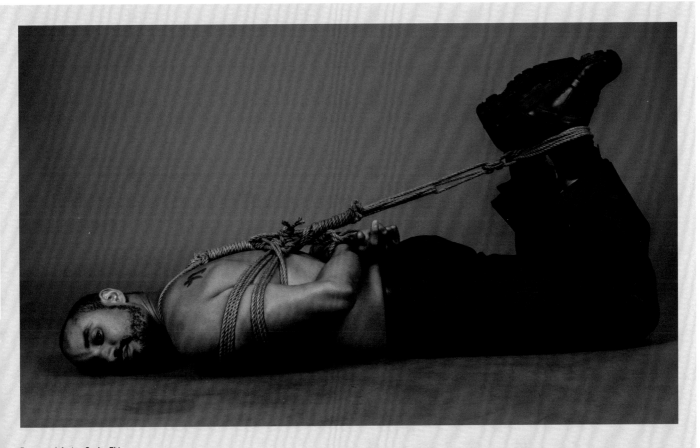

Downward-facing Gyaku Ebi

Wrap a whole lot

In this variation, use up your extra rope by wrapping a lot around the series of lines that ran from the ankles to the chest. Split the bundle of lines apart and tuck the ends between those lines to keep it from unraveling. This tie can be challenging on the neck. Leave enough wiggle room so that your partner can get their head from side to side. For longer scenes, a pillow is also a kindness to the body.

6

Ebi or Kuri (Shrimp or Ball Tie)

The Shrimp or Ball Tie (also known as Kuri which translates as "chestnut") starts with the Bottom sitting cross-legged, though more flexible Bottoms can sit in lotus position. After the chest is attached to the ankles, it is possible (as shown) to lower the Bottom onto her back or side. Please remember to support the Bottom's upper body and head as you change her position; tipping her over without support may lead to head or shoulder trauma.

This pose was originally designed as a torture position because of the breathing challenges created by diaphragm pressure. It is hard to get a full breath of air when in Ebi. Because of this chance of positional asphyxia, make sure to keep an eye on your partner in this position, and be ready to release them when needed.

One of the great things about this position is that you can modify it so easily for a variety of body types. Instead of wrapping around the back of the neck, you can pull down taking the line through the chest harness. You can pull down just to the comfort of your Bottom. The choice is also there to make the tie tight and extreme. Experiment, and have fun!

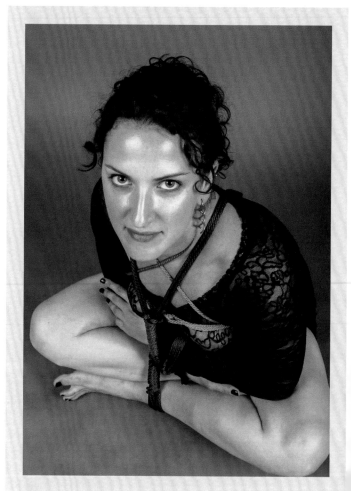

Finished Upright Ball Tie

Tie a chest harness

In this case, I chose to use a **Halter Top Harness** (see page 67). The more classical Ebi begins with a **Box Tie** (see page 61), and thus skips **steps 2 and 3.**

1

Tie both wrists in front

Fingertips to elbow on each side, folded in front of the chest, bind the arms using a **Two-Column Tie** (see page 38).

2

Attach the wrists to the chest harness

Wrap the long end of the leftover line around the center of the chest harness, then bring the lines in back to tie off.

3

Bind both ankles

Have the Bottom fold her ankles in front of her, sitting cross-legged. Then, tie the two ankles as if they were a single column (see page 34), with all the knots above the ankles.

4

Wrap around the back of the neck

If you choose to have the Ebi tie tuck underneath the chest harness in front, it avoids pressure on the neck. This changes the type of breathing compression and difficulty.

5

Make a lark's head

Tuck the ends through the bight from the one-column tie.

6

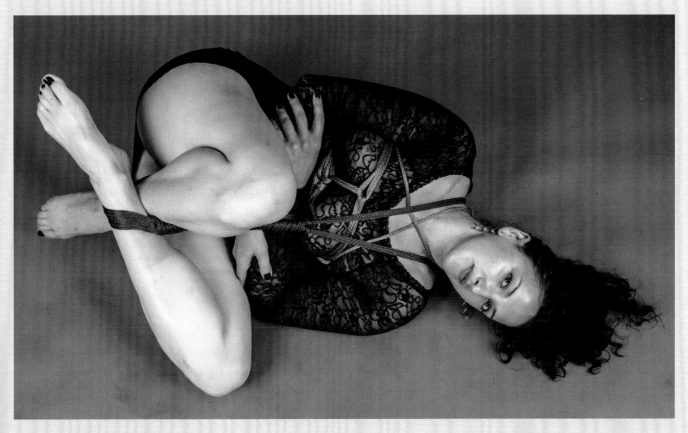

Finished Laying Ball Tie

Cinch down chest to ankles

Pull the chest towards the ankles by putting tension on the lark's head. Then, tie off with an overhand knot. Now, you could either just sit back and enjoy, or, supporting both the head and the body of the Bottom, tip her on her side to expose her for your amusement (or to adjust tension on her body). Adding pillows under her legs, shoulder and neck can also affect body comfort. Some find these changes in tension and pose will allow them to stay bound for longer.

7

Chair Tie

A true classic of "Western" bondage (a favorite of "cops and robbers" movies and abduction scenes), the Chair Tie consists of four **Two-Column Ties** (see page 38). Though technically simple, it can be visually alluring and erotic.

To further dive into the Western theme of bondage (and that "damsel in distress" concept), there are additional elements that can be delicious to include:

- Using white rope.
- Gagging them with a bandana or other piece of fabric, tied around the back of their head. Make sure your partner does not have any jaw issues (such as TMJ) before you gag them.
  - Using simple blindfolds.
  - Playing dress-up.
  - Role-playing "bad guy" and "good guy" roles.

But don't think this tie is just for the ladies. Using this tie on men exposes their genitals for special attention, and puts a nice twist on the theme. Chair Ties can be good fun for everyone.

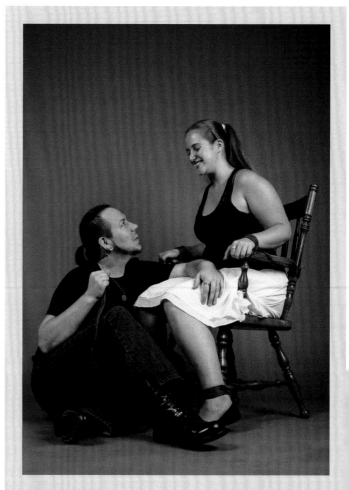

Tying a Chair Tie

Find a sturdy chair

Use a chair with four legs and an open back, multi-column back, sturdy armrests or some other style with openings in it. A struggling Bottom has the chance of injuring themselves or accidentally destroying a flimsy chair.

1

Tie wrists to chair back

Using a **Two-Column Tie** (see page 38), tie the left wrist to the outermost left column on the chair. In this case, we used the armrests. Repeat on the right side.

2

Tie ankles to chair legs

Use a **Two-Column Tie** to attach the left ankle to the left forward chair leg. Repeat on the right side. If there is some sort of support bar between the chair legs, tie above the support to stop the ankle ties from slipping off if the Bottom tips the chair backwards.

3

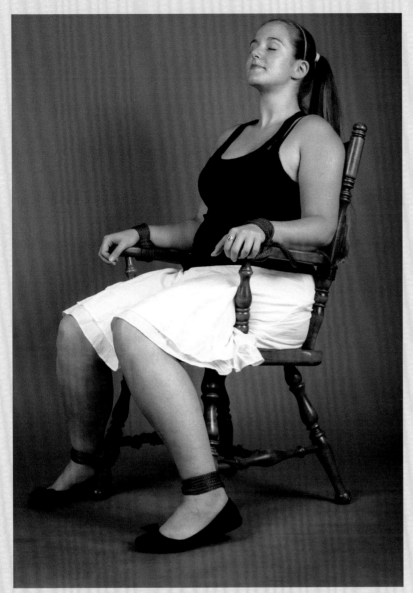

Wrap a lot

Get rid of the excess rope however makes you happiest.

The one major problem with Chair Ties is that fidgety Bottoms can try to escape and, in doing so, knock the chair over. I recommend propping the chair against a wall or keeping an eye on Bottoms so they do not accidentally hurt themselves.

4

Finished Chair Tie

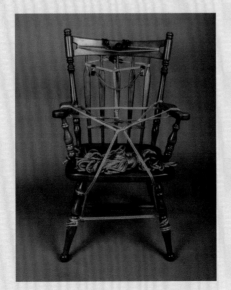

That's not quite what we meant...

but it would be a fun way to practice!

Kani (Crab) and Niwatori (Little Chicken)

A classical application of the **Two-Column Tie** (see page 38), the Kani pose has two basic positions for the Bottom to be in: on their knees or sitting down with their legs in front of them. Other options—having the Bottom lay on his back, side or stomach—are all just variations of these first two ideas. The pose can be modified for those whose ankles do not touch their thighs by using a **Spread Two-Column** variation (see page 41).

The "Little Chicken" pose is created by attaching the wrist to the upper arm, using the same tie. Try tying the knots on the back side of the arm to avoid the chance of the Bottom untying the ropework with their teeth. With Niwatori, arms can also be bound in front of the body, or behind the back, using the loose ends of the two-column ties to lash the arms into place.

Be careful of the sensitive skin at the back of the knees and elbows! As you push the rope through, make sure your nails don't catch the skin and that the line is pulled slowly. The inside of the knee and elbow are a horrible place for rope burn.

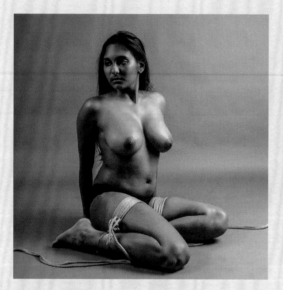
Kani kneeling

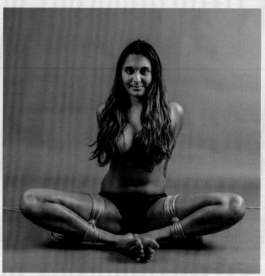
Kani with knees spread

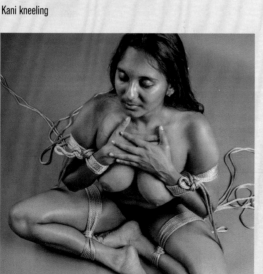
Niwatori in front

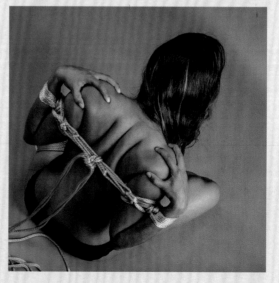
Niwatori bound back

Ankle to Wrist

This simple tie is comprised of two sets of **Two-Column Ties** (see page 38). Each set is one ankle tied to one wrist. I usually tie this pose with the Bottom sitting down, and then roll them onto their back or side after they are tied. Remember, when moving a bound Bottom, support their weight to avoid shoulder, hip, back, and head injuries.

Some Bottoms prefer to have their back cushioned on a bed and then lift their limbs up in the air to be bound. Having additional support can help a lot when trying to get frisky in your bondage, or when trying to use this tie with the chest down, one shoulder down on the ground, and ass up in the air.

While playing with a partner, try moving between positions and combinations without getting someone completely out of rope. In this case, you can untie the left ankle from its corresponding wrist, and take that rope (or a new one), and use it to tie a **One-Column Tie** (see page 34) around the exposed left wrist. You can now tie that wrist down to a bed, or over to the space between the right ankle and wrist to create something all new!

Keeping the ties going can be engaging for some Bottoms and Tops, while others enjoy staying in only one pose for an entire scene. Check in with each other as you go, and/or before you play, to make sure everyone gets their needs and desires met.

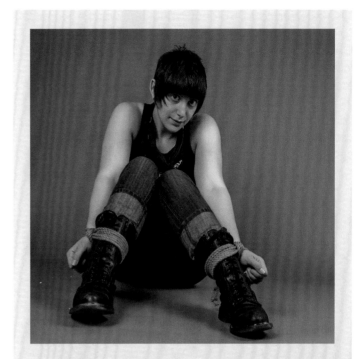

Seated Ankle to Wrist

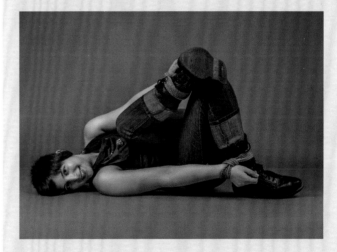

Laying with Ankle to Wrist

Captive Tie

Also referred to as Kotobu Ryo-tekubi, which means "binding both hands at the back of the head," the Captive Tie can be done either playfully or in an intense manner. For something more sensual, caress their body as you lift their hands overhead, moving slowly with each step. If you enjoy being rough, after you have carefully lifted their arms into place, pull your Bottom close and firmly wrap each line with a sense of determination.

Since the hands are pulled overhead, some Bottoms may be quick to lose circulation; make sure to squeeze their hands regularly. If they go numb, untie the waist line and move their hands below their heart.

This bondage can be done with one piece of rope (if using a **Two-Column Tie**) or two (for the more lenient **Spread Two-Column Variation**), and is shown here with two pieces of line. The option shown here is considered a more lenient version.

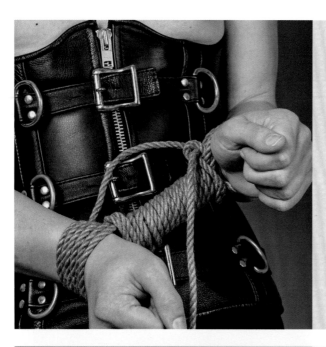

Bind hands

Using a **Two-Column Tie** (see page 38) or **Spread Two-Column Tie** (see page 41), attach the wrists to each other in front of the body.

1

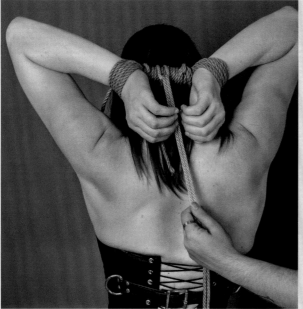

Run line from wrists to back of waist

Carefully lift the hands overhead, and then pull them down behind the head. As you lift the arms overhead, the elbows will spread out and the wrist tie will get tighter. Make sure to go slowly and check in to make sure you do not strain a wrist or shoulder of your Bottom. If you are using two pieces of rope, this is the point where you would add your second piece before running the line down, as shown here.

2

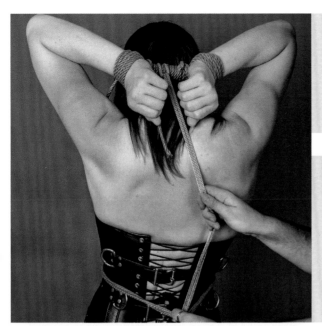

Wrap around waist

Wrap the folded line around the waist.

3

Create lark's head

When you return to the center of the back, you will see that by wrapping the torso, you have created an area that rope can be tucked through. Pull the ends through this open space, then pull back in the direction you came from.

4

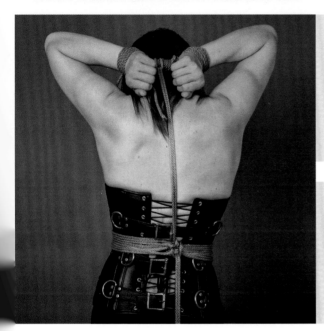

Wrap a second time and make a lark's head

Lay the second set of lines below the first set. When you come back to the first lark's head, you will see that by wrapping a second time, you have created a new loop that rope can be tucked through. Pull the ends through this loop, then pull up and back the direction the line came from.

5

Repeat steps 4 and 5 twice more

Wrap just below the other wraps, around the waist. Tuck ends through the newest loop and pull in the direction the line came from. Wrap a fourth time, just below the third wrap, tuck the ends through the newest loop and pull in the direction that line came from.

6

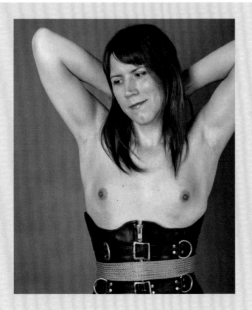

Tie off

Hold the rope 2 inches (5 cm) above the waist line using your left hand and let the ends drop down. Take the loose ends and tuck them up under all of the wraps of the waist line, pulling the ends through the loop that was just created. Pull the half hitch you have just created tight.

Finished Captive Tie

7

Rope Corsets and Erotic Macramé

Having tackled the basics of Japanese-style rope bondage, let's look at a category of ties inspired by Shibari—Erotic Macramé. This category of rope bondage is a blend of Japanese-inspired rope bondage, macramé, and rope as fashion.

One of the most striking uses for erotic macramé is the rope corset. Ever noticed how expensive corsets are? Now you can make your own for a fraction of the cost. This design of rope corset allows for the creation of wide variety of styles once you have these basic concepts down.

In this chapter, we will cover the following applications:

- Basic Rope Corset
- Double Spine Rope Corset
- Fancy Rope Corsets
- Rope Gauntlets
- Gauntlet Bondage

You can make rope corsets as fancy or simple as you like them. Every single time you apply a rope corset, it will be slightly different. No two rope corsets are quite the same. This is not a flaw, but an opportunity to show that you spent the time and energy to make this one unique.

If you are interested, you can also break out your old macramé books from the 1970s or modern survivalist books on para-cord tying to get your knotty self going at any point with these techniques. Try combining these patterns with the ideas presented here   and find your own approach to rope corsets.

Watch out for your partner's breathing as you use corsets, as the restriction of the diaphragm affects some Bottoms quickly, and others over time. Keep in mind that if it took you 20 minutes to craft a corset, it will take 10-20 minutes to untie it. Have those emergency scissors around just in case, and encourage the Bottom to sit as the Top calmly unties in such situations.

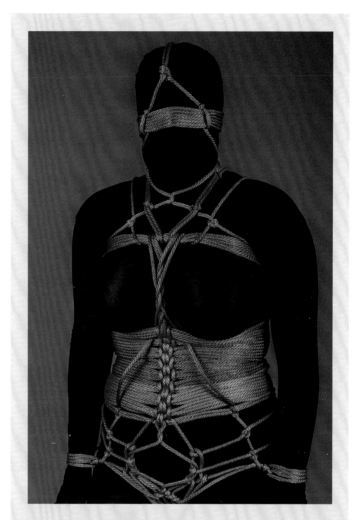

An Exposed Cherry Crotch Rope (page 102) and Double Spine Rope Corset (page 90) can be combined for a dramatic effect.

Basic Rope Corset

Basic Rope Corsets are essentially a series of lark's heads down the torso. By learning to construct this classical form, you will begin developing the skills needed for more advanced variations. In this version, the spine of lark's heads is down the center front of the torso, but the same design and technique can allow you to have the spine down the center back or side of the corset. Keeping the rope spine straight is the key to this pattern.

When crafting rope corsets, mixing media allows for alternating colors, shine, and texture. Material diversity can be quite eye-catching. On the other hand, using all one type of rope creates the visual of a more classic fabric corset. Try making both styles, and see what appeals more to you and your partner.

This rope corset is constructed using four total pieces of 25-30ft (8-10 meter) MFP and jute rope.

Identify column

Choose a column. The most common column for rope corsets is the torso, but as you will see further in this chapter, almost any column will do. In the case of torsos, keep an eye out for rigging challenges such as additional midsection curves, bruises and spinal protrusions. Some bodies are not suited to long rope corsets—consider building a rope cincher or belt instead.

1

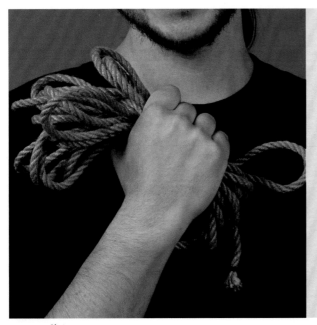

Find your rope

The easiest length of rope to work with is 25-40ft (8-12 meters) in length. Anything longer than this may get tangled as you weave back and forth, and with anything shorter, you will be splicing on additional pieces every other wrap. By using multiple pieces of rope, the option is present to create colorful patterns. You are welcome to use longer ropes with these points in mind.

2

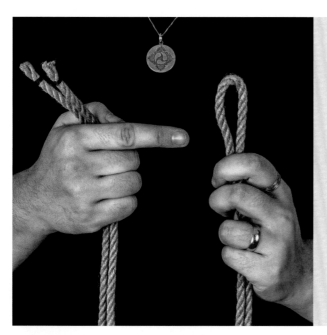

Find the bight

Fold your rope in half and hold the rope by the bight.

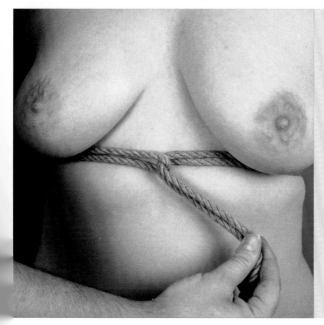

Wrap and create lark's head

With the bight located at the front center of the torso, wrap the doubled line around the torso with the ropes just under the breasts or pectoral mass. Pull the ends through the bight, then pull the ends back in the direction that they came from to create reverse tension. The lines around the torso should be snug but not restrictive.

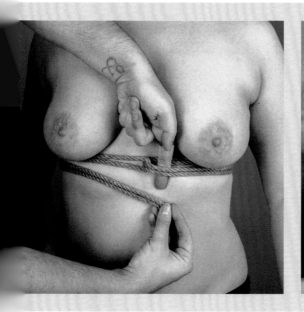

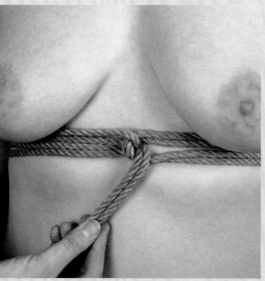

Create second lark's head

Lay the second set of lines below the first set. When you come back to the first lark's head, you will see that by wrapping a second time, you have created a new loop that rope can be tucked through. Pull the ends through this loop, then pull up and back in the direction the line came from.

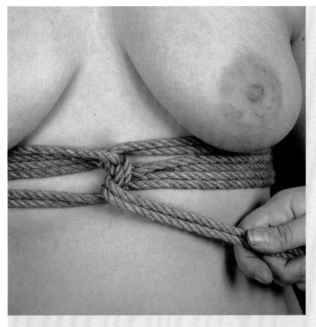

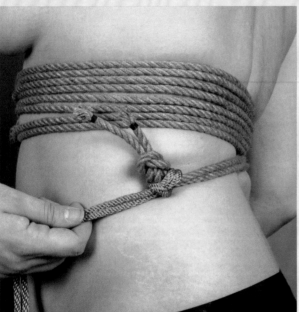

Repeat step 5 until you run out of rope

Wrap just below the last line. Make sure to keep tension even with each line, and straighten the spine of lark's heads that form at the center of the torso.

Any time you run out of rope, **add rope** (see page 53).

6

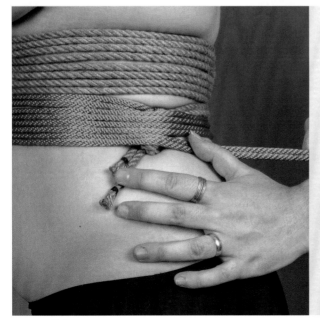

Continue until you reach the bottom of the corset

Continue to wrap lines in alternating directions while maintaining a straight spine of lark's heads at the center of the torso and even tension on each wrap. Pause every few lines to make sure the lines are touching at the side and that you are covering up any knots from adding new rope by laying lines over the knots to conceal them. The corset has reached the bottom when it looks right to you.

7

Tie off wraps

When you reach the end of your corset, split the two lines in your hand. One will go through the bight at the base of the corset, just as if you were about to do an additional wrap. Create a square knot by going left over right, then right over left. Tuck the ends of the square knot underneath the base of the corset.

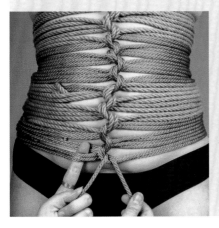 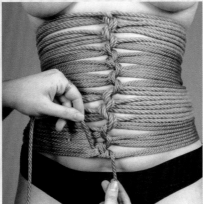 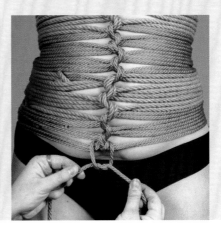

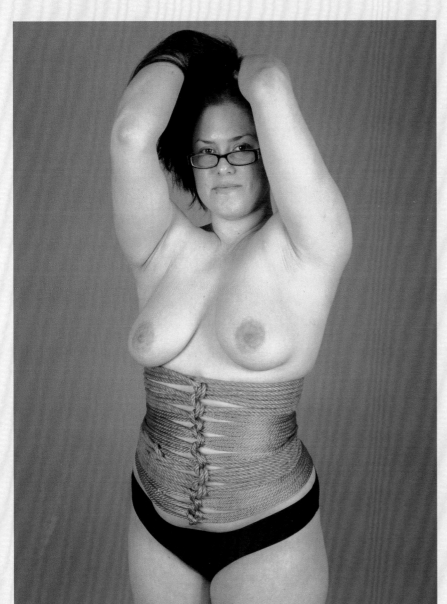

Finished **Basic Rope Corset**

Double Spine Rope Corset

The primary complaint about the **Basic Rope Corset** is that lines of rope will compact upon one another with movement, no matter the size of the person you are tying. This variation addresses part of this issue by anchoring the layers of lines at the front and back of each line, not just at one point on each wrap. Additional spines can be added as desired, creating even more support and stability.

But take note—each time an additional spine is added, the rope corset will get tighter. Have a pair of EMT shears available just in case the corseted person needs to get out fast.

This specific corset was built using four 25-30ft (8-10 meter) pieces of jute, and 1 piece of 25-30ft (8-10 meter) MFP.

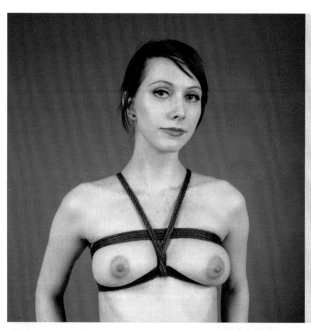

Build harness

Create the **Basic Chest Harness** (see page 46). This corset is an extension of that tie.

1

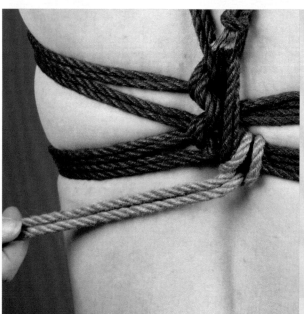

Attach lark's head to Main Body

Attach a new piece of line (see page 53) to the center back of the chest harness. For dramatic effect, this is an opportunity to change colors of rope or textures of line, though staying with the same width of line is encouraged.

2

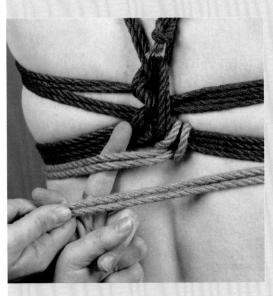 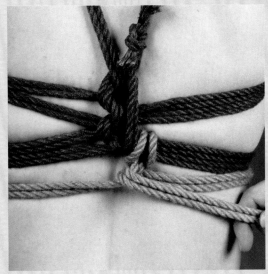

Wrap torso under chest harness and create lark's head

Wrap directly underneath the chest harness. Once you have returned to the center back, pull the ends up through the newly created gap on the back, then pull down and back in the direction the line came from.

3

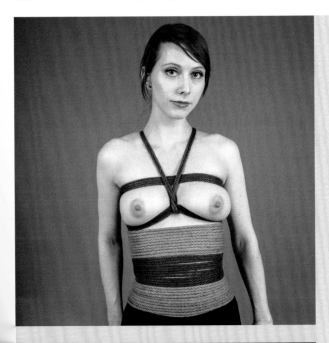

Wrap around torso and create repeating lark's heads

Lay the second set of lines below the first set. When you come back to the first lark's head of the corset segment, you will see that by wrapping a second time, you have created a new loop that rope can be tucked up through, just as you did with the **Chest Harness** or **Basic Rope Corset**. Maintain even tension as you repeat this pattern, straightening the spine of the corset down the back towards the rump as you go.

Each time you run out of rope, **add more rope** (see page 53). Changing colors creates drama, or use all one tone and texture for a continuous look. Pause every few lines to make sure that the lines are touching at the side and that you are covering up any knots from adding new rope by laying lines over the knots to conceal them. When you reach the bottom of the corset, tie off the line with step 8 from the **Basic Rope Corset** (see page 86).

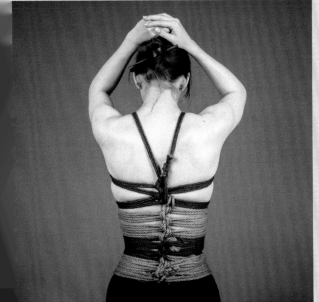

4

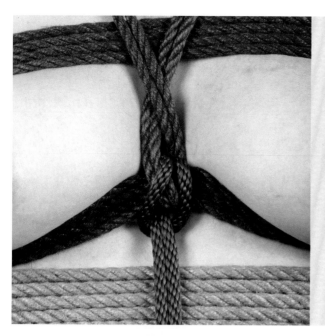

Attach lark's head to center

Attach a new rope (see page 53) to the center front of the chest harness. For dramatic effect, this is an opportunity to change colors of rope or textures of line, though staying with the same width of line is preferable for a more classically attractive rope corset.

5

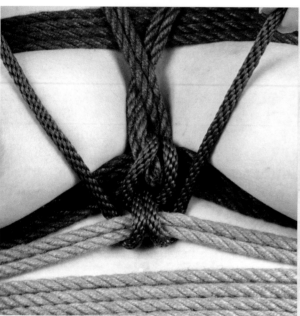

Begin laying second spine

Lay the doubled line over the first two lines of the corset. Tuck each end up underneath the first two lines of the corset, one on each side of the spine that is being built.

6

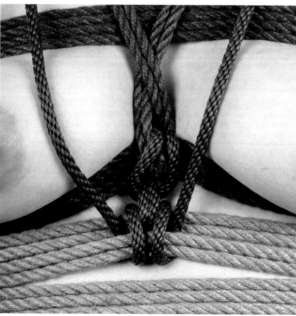

Create center pattern

Lay the separated spine line over the next two wraps of the corset. Tuck each end up underneath the previous wrap.

7

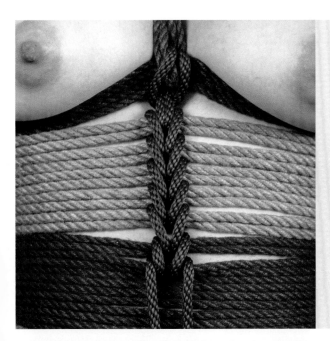

Continue herringbone spine

Repeat this two sets down and one set up pattern, making sure to keep the spine that is being set in a straight line down the center front of the torso.

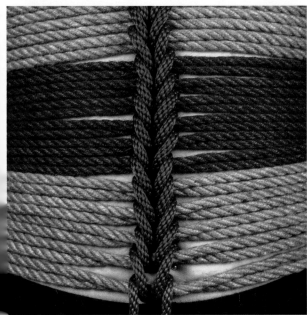

Tie off

By the bottom of the corset you with have an elegant herringbone-patterned spine down the center front of the torso. Tie off the ends of the rope with a square knot or other technique, and do lots of wraps or twists to use up the remaining rope.

Fancy Rope Corsets

Is the **Double Spine Rope Corset** not ornate enough for you? Perhaps you want to design something truly unique for a party, or want to weave a very restrictive design on your lover to control their posture (remember those EMT shears!).

Here I have done additional looping with a single blue line back up the torso in a diagonal pattern on each side of the front center spine. Having reached the top, each single line was taken over a shoulder, tied off to the back of the chest harness, and then brought around to the front to pull the lines off the clavicle.

Additional ideas include:

- Adding spines on each side of the corset
- Creating diamonds by looping in different directions
- Making multi-media art by doing all decoration with ribbon, fabric, latex stripping, thin line, plastic, or silk cording
- Corseting down the entire body for hobble skirts or rope mummification
- Weaving spirals, loops, hearts (see page 25), and other patterns into the lines
- Finding inspiration from a wide variety of macramé or fiber craft books

Go out and have fun, and see where you can create rope corsets. Let your creativity fly!

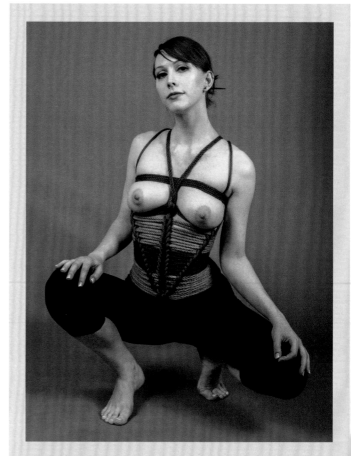

Finished Diagonal Pattern Corset

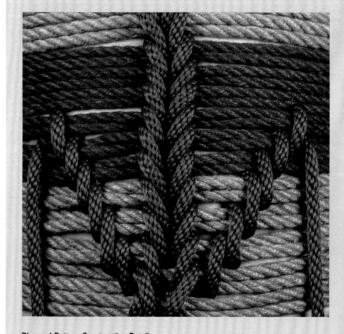

Diagonal Pattern Construction Detail

Rope Gauntlets

Who says that rope corsets can only be woven on the torso? Rope Gauntlets are a great way to wear rope to a fetish party that can then be taken off to tie up a delicious morsel—or be a practical fashion accessory for anyone who enjoys erotic wrestling. Follow the steps in the **Basic Rope Corset**, starting at the wrist with a slightly loose wrap.

Build up the arms with repeating lark's heads, and tie off with a half hitch when you run out of rope. Tuck the loose ends underneath the bondage to create a smooth line. Repeat on the other arm. Combining a pair of rope gauntlets with head bondage or a corset belt can create a very sexy and intimidating look, as shown in Chapter 1 (see page 23). It is also a great way for a Top to carry around their rope at a party!

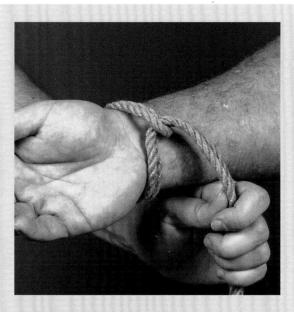

Beginning the Gauntlets

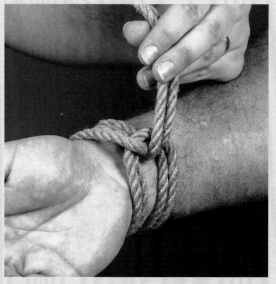

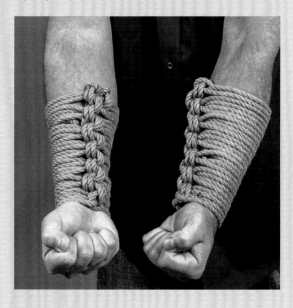

Finished Gauntlets

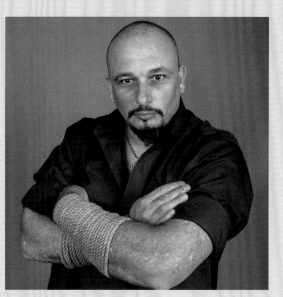

Gauntlet Bondage

Rope corsets can also be used as a form of restraint. Create a corset around two legs, two forearms, or run a corset around the waist and both arms at the same time. In this example forearms have been corseted together to finish the bound look with a **Fancy Rope Corset.**

Make sure to not tie off on only one loop or strand of the gauntlet bondage, lest the gauntlets keep tightening down from the pressure. If you want to attach the Gauntlet Bondage to other pieces of equipment or bound bodies, try sliding rope underneath three or four of the sets of rope before coming back up, enabling pressure distribution. Gauntlet Bondage can also be a lot of fun making a corset around two people's torsos at once.

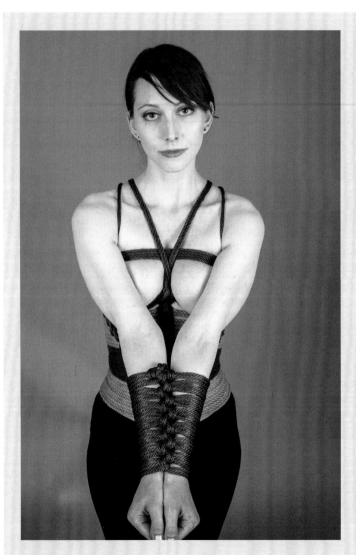
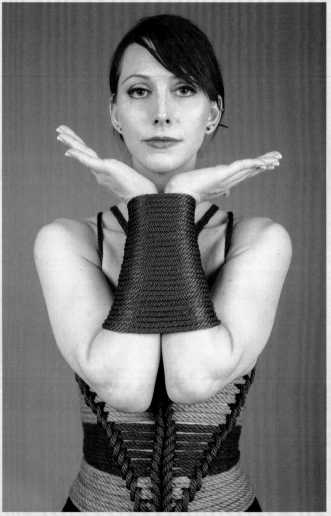

Crotch Ropes

Having bound the torso, wrists, ankles, arms, and pretty much everything else... we need to make sure to learn how to tie one last segment of the body—the genital region. Call it whatever you like—loins, groin, down there, forbidden fruit—it's an area of the body that many individuals, for a variety of reasons, enjoy having rope on.

Some of those reasons include:

- Direct genital stimulation
- Body decoration to enhance attractiveness
- Having hand-holds to grab onto during sex
- Tie-points for attaching wrist and ankle cuffs
- Sensual touch and sensation play
- Constant awareness of a lover's presence

With all of these delightful reasons to choose from (and likely more that you can think of), each person who ties crotch ropes or wears them will make them their own. These forms of ropework come in a variety of styles, each with their own pros and cons, but we will focus on three styles in this book:

- Basic Crotch Rope
- Exposing the Cherry
- Strap-On Harness

Are there options out there for these kinds of play made out of other materials? Absolutely! It's fun to try out lots of different approaches to crotch play. But leather is a porous material that can carry bodily fluids and transmit some viruses, and PVC harnesses have to be bought for only the person who will be wearing them. Gain or lose any weight, and you have to buy a new one. Tying a crotch harness out of rope (whether for sex-play or decoration) allows it to fit perfectly for today, and be modified for the person wearing them. How fun!

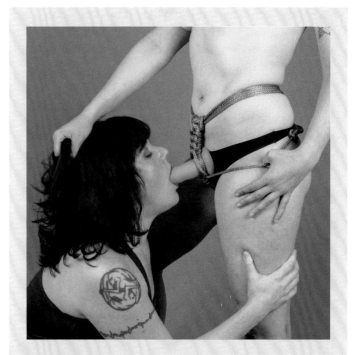

Crotch ropes and Strap-on Harnesses can be a lot of fun... just make sure to wash them afterwards (see page 28).

Basic Crotch Rope

Also known as Matanawa (tying the groin), the Basic Crotch Rope can be a lot of fun, a great way to restrict access to the genitals, a lovely decorative detail, or a way to stimulate the clitoris or anus.

Almost any sort of rope is usable for a crotch rope, however I suggest using MFP or some sort of soft, washable line. For more advanced players, hemp, jute and other natural fibers are worth exploring—unless

someone has an allergy of course. Having a Bottom bring their own rope for this tie allows for ease in keeping straight which ropes need to be cleaned, and letsthe Bottom determine what type of texture they want on their genital region.

For this basic tie, I use 15-30ft (5-10 meters) of line, depending on the size of the individual being bound and how intricate I want to decorate after the base structure is on.

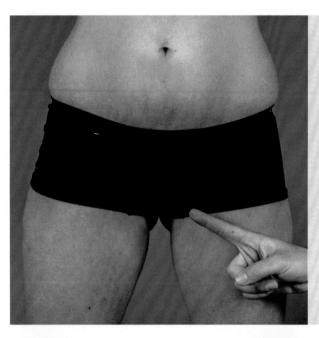

Identify crotch

Choose a crotch. Identify anything that might require modifications to the tie, such as external genitals, piercings, or body hair. Just because someone has piercings does not mean you can't tie a crotch rope on them; you just need to be careful doing anything quickly, or you may choose to tie an **Exposing the Cherry** tie instead (see page 102).

1

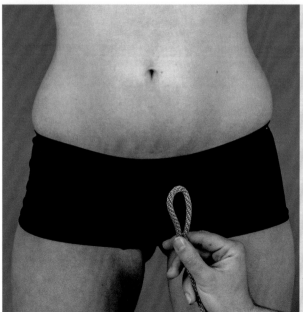

Find your rope bight

Having chosen your rope, fold the line in half.
Hold the rope by the bight.

2

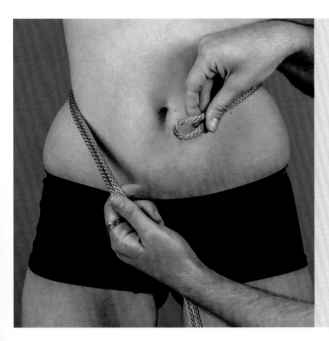

Wrap torso at waistline

With the bight located just below the belly button, wrap the folded line around the torso with the ropes at the waistline. On individuals with rounded waists or with extra curves, consider wrapping under the belly, just above the hips.

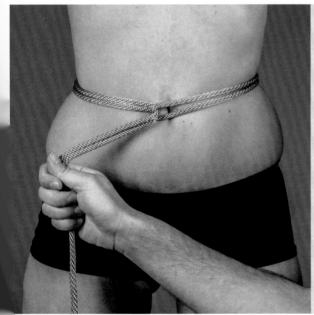

Create lark's head

By pulling the ends through the bight, create a lark's head. Pull the ends through the bight, then pull the ends back in the direction that they came from, placing tension on the lines. The lines around the waist should be snug but not restrictive.

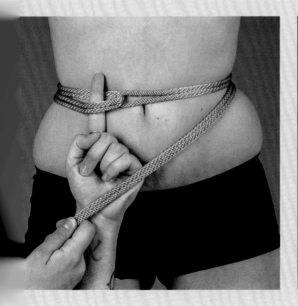

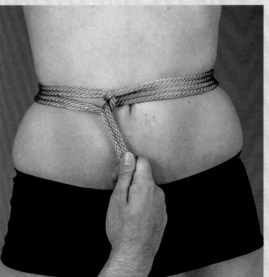

Create second lark's head

Lay the second set of lines just below the first set, pulling in the opposite direction of the first. When you come back to the first lark's head, you will see that by wrapping a second time, you have created a new loop that rope can be tucked through. Pull the ends up through this loop, then pull down.

Tie off wraps

Using a half hitch, tie off around all of the waist lines. Pull tight.

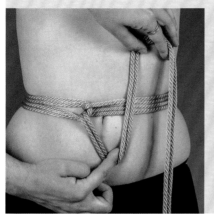 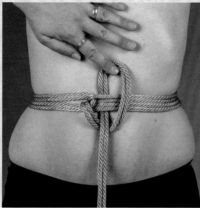 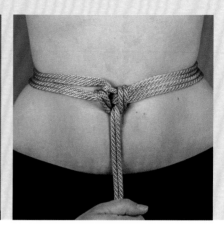

6

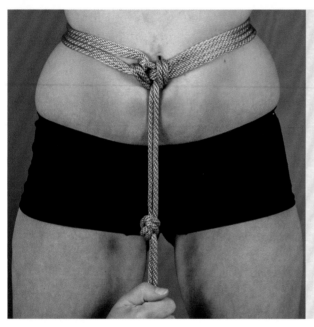

Tie an over-hand knot

Many individuals enjoy having a knot placed appropriately to stimulate the clitoris, anus, vaginal opening, or perineum (the soft region between the groin and the anus). Ask the person you are binding what would appeal to them. This step is optional if you or your partner are not interested in additional sensation, or find such knots uncomfortable. You can also tie a series of knots to stimulate a variety of points, hold in plugs, or to deny access to the region.

7

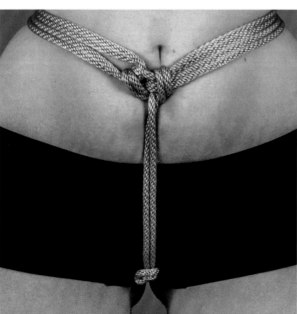

Pull line through the legs

Make the line snug, but not painful. If working with individuals with external genitals, split the line apart as you place the line to avoid painful compression.

8

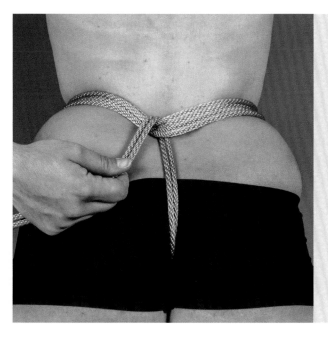

Tuck underneath waist line

Having run the doubled line through the legs, tuck it underneath all of the waist lines at the center of the back.

9

Tie off line

Using a half hitch knot, tie off around the line that came up between the legs.

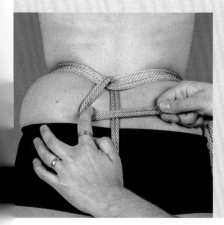 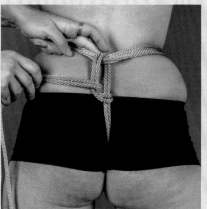 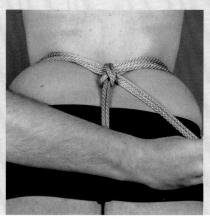

10

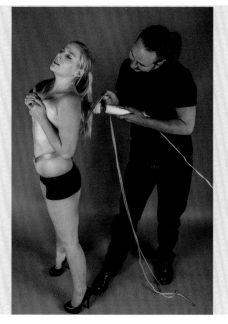

Once the line is tied off, you can do a wide variety of things with the leftover rope. Add decorative details. Begin a rope corset. Tie the line to a chest harness for a forced wedgie. Or, in this case, we chose to leave the line loose and use it to transmit vibrations. Rope transmits vibrations from your favorite vibrator, and natural fibers work even better than synthetic fibers.

Exposing the Cherry

Though many people enjoy the sensation of a crotch rope, what do you do if you want to gain access to what the crotch rope is covering up? Perhaps the rope has been rubbing the delicate skin too much, or you want to enjoy penetration after enjoying the **Basic Crotch Rope** for a while. Maybe you like the idea of being artistic, or binding around the ass itself. If Sakura (another pseudonym for a crotch rope) is to bind the "cherry," then this is to "expose the cherry."

It is easier to split apart the crotch rope if no knots are tied in the central line. You can expose the groin even if there are over-hand knots tied, but less will be exposed than would be if no knots were involved. Thus, if you know you will be splitting the lines later in a scene, consider skipping step 7 when tying the **Basic Crotch Rope.**

Follow steps 1-10 of the **Basic Crotch Rope** (page 98) before moving on to steps below.

Construct Basic Crotch Rope

Follow steps 1-10 of the **Basic Crotch Rope** (page 98).

You can play for hours with a **Basic Crotch Rope**, and when ready to gain access to the nether regions, begin the steps below. The version shown below is shown with the knot.

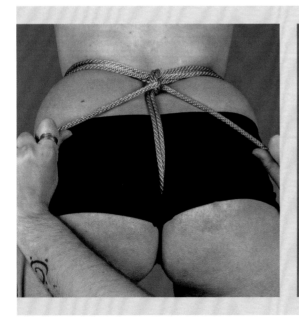

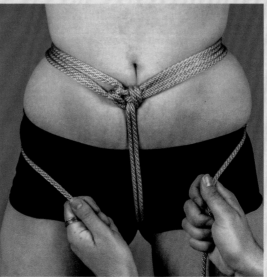

Split the lines

Take one line in each hand. Pull both of the lines to the front, running one line along the hip on each side of the rump.

11

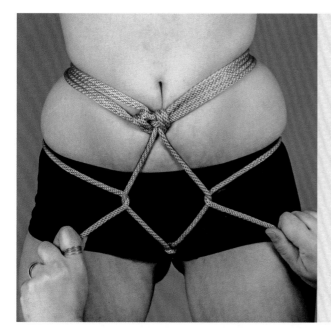

Pull ends underneath center front crotch rope

Pull ends underneath center front crotch rope. On the right side, take the line and tuck it underneath the right strand of the crotch rope. Repeat on the left side. Pull both lines snug, but not uncomfortably so.

12

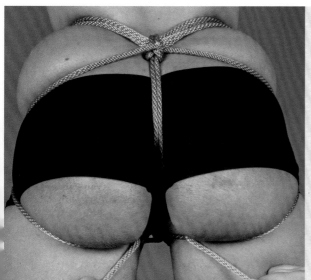

Pull both the lines to the back

Run one line along the lower hip on each side of the rump. On the right side, take the line and tuck it underneath the right strand of the crotch rope at the base of the ass. Repeat on the left side. Pull both lines snug, but not uncomfortably so. In doing so, you have exposed the "cherry."

13

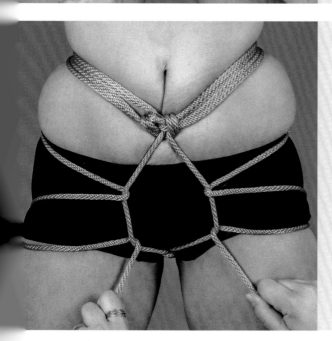

Pull ends underneath center front crotch rope

Run one line along the lower hip on each side of the rump, immediately below the last hip line. On the right side, take the line and tuck it underneath the right strand of the forward crotch rope just below the last hip line. Repeat on the left side.

14

Tie off lines

Lay the right line over the lower right hip line. Tie off using a half hitch. Repeat on the left side using the left line.

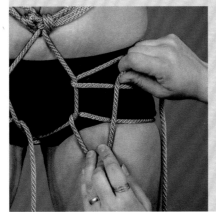 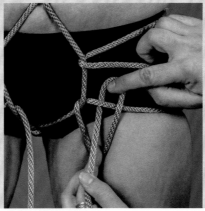 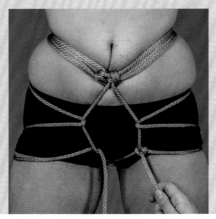

15

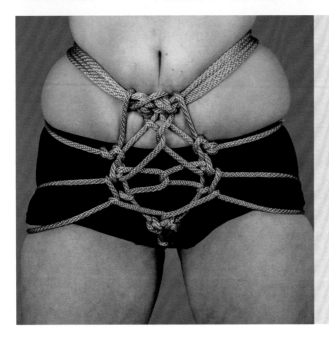

Wrap a whole lot

Take the ends and wrap them around something. In this spider-web pattern, lines were crossed over each other and caught at each side of the open diamond from the initial tie. Any rigging at this point is purely for decorative value, as the structure of the tie was finished at step 15. This concept is sometimes referred to as kazari-nawa, the use of excess rope to decorate a tie that has been completed.

16

Strap-On Harness

Whether looking for a fun sex toy or enjoying gender-bending role-playing, the Strap-on Harness is a way to attach a dildo to the pelvis in a secure manner. Tested and modified over years of exploration in the swinger communities and beyond, this harness was designed with a variety of body types and sizes in mind, and provides opportunities for use whether you already have external genitals or not.

For those of you who have never had a "cock" strapped on before, before you begin, hold the dildo in your hand and place it on top of your pelvis. What feels right for your center of gravity and how you thrust? This information will be used in step 14.

To begin, follow steps 1-9, except step 7, of the **Basic Crotch Rope** (see page 98), using a 25-40ft (8-12 meter) length of machine-washable rope.

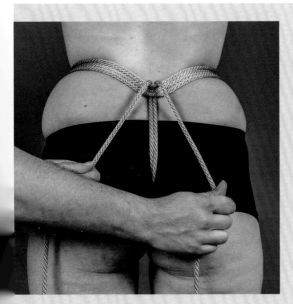
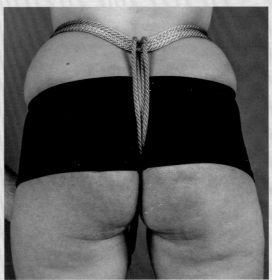

Pull line back through legs

Split the line apart and run the lines back through the legs, one on each side of the initial crotch rope.

10

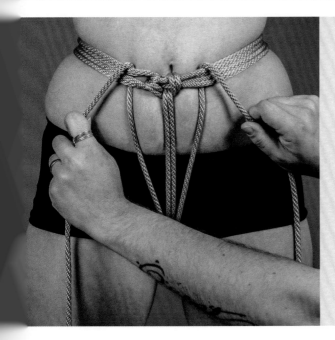

Tuck underneath front of waist line

Having run the doubled line through the legs, tuck it underneath all of the waist lines at the center of the front, one on each side of the original crotch line.

11

Tie half hitch knot right

Lay the right line across all four of the crotch ropes, and tie a half hitch around them.
The half hitch should not include the left active line. Pull the line snug and tighten down knot.

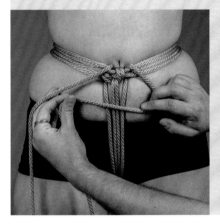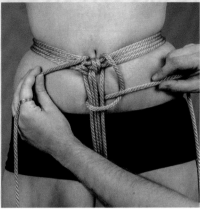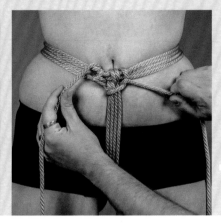

12

Tie half hitch knot left

Lay the left line across all four of the crotch ropes, and tie a half hitch around them.
The half hitch should not include the right active line. Pull the line snug and tighten down knot.

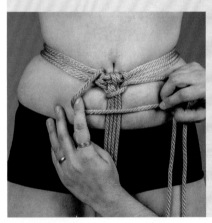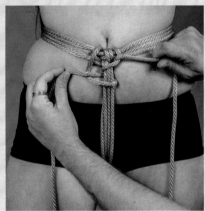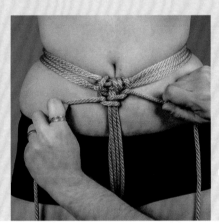

13

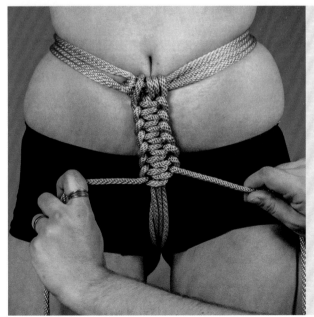

Repeat steps 12 and 13

Repeat half hitch knots 2-15 times on each side until you reach the point where the top of your dildo should rest. Use what feels right on the body that will be supporting your attached "cock."

For individuals with a biological penis, it is usually easier to have the dildo rest directly above your biological equipment. This series of half hitches stabilizes the dildo, but may also act as additional stimulation for your partner in some positions.

14

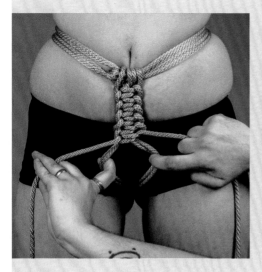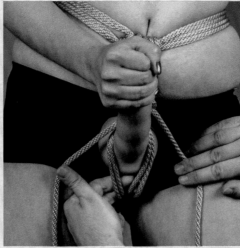

Split lines and slide in dildo

Two lines will lie on each side of your "cock." Using a dildo with a flared/flange base is recommended, since non-flange dildos have more likelihood of slipping out during active play.

15

Tie half hitch knots below dildo

As you tie the knots, make sure to snug them up to the base of the "cock" to make sure it does not slip out.

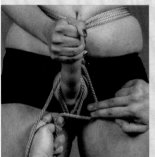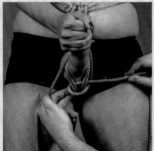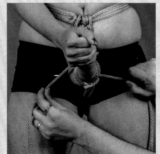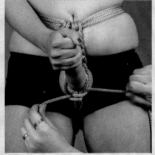

16

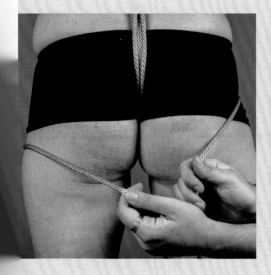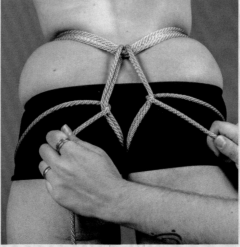

Pull both the lines to the back and rear under crotch rope

Run one line along the lower hip on each side of the rump. This placement of line can also be done under the ass-cheek, as it was done while **Exposing the Cherry** (see page 102). On the right side, take the line and tuck it underneath the two right strands of the crotch. Repeat on the left side. Pull both lines snug, but not uncomfortably so.

17

Tie off lines

Take the right line and tie a half hitch around the right two strands of the crotch rope. Repeat with the left line.

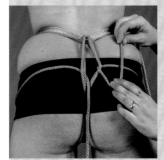 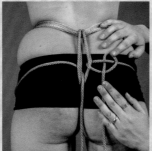 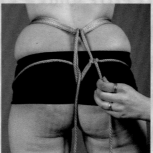 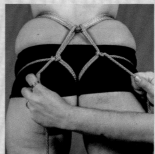

18

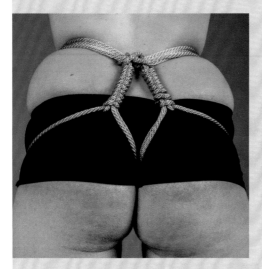 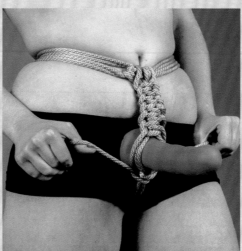

Wrap a whole lot

If there is any rope left over, wrap around the waist lines, weave up and down around the hips, or use up the rope in any other way you find aesthetically appealing. Your finished product? A strap on harness that is machine washable, fits you every time, and does not wobble from side to side. If during play the harness loosens up, just untie those final wraps and snug down the hip lines… and keep having fun.

19

Play responsibly and have fun!

Remember that some dildos are made of silicone and are thus easily cleanable, but others are made of porous rubbers and "mystery materials." You can slide a condom on these toys for enjoying them without worrying about bacteria or other concerns.

When playing with strap-on harnesses, lube is also important for a variety of orifices. Too much lube is better than not enough! Water-based lubricants are a great choice, though some folks prefer silicone lube if their dildo is not made of silicone. Oil-based lubes break down condoms and are thus not a great choice for this sort of play.

Enjoy your crotch-ropes... and all of the kinds of bondage you have learned! Make it your own, and come back to this book over and over again for instructions, inspiration, and a little bit of titillation too.

Where Do We Go From Here?

Now you know the basic secrets of Japanese style rope bondage:

- Fold your rope in half
- There are only a few knots, and they are pretty easy
- More complicated ties are usually just layers or combinations of basic ties
- Enjoying the type of bondage that you and your partner enjoy is important
- Being present and in the moment matters
- Communication is key

So, where do we go from here?

For some people, pulling out this book from time to time and having fun with the basics is perfect. For others, you will want to buy some more books to diversify your knowledge. You might be interested in finding other people into rope bondage to learn with or play with. Perhaps you want to be inspired (and turned on) by the work of others through erotic photography, rope performances, and pornography. Or… you might to just want to go buy some rope.

Options for all of these are listed in the following pages. Remember as you explore that each person is on their own path with rope work. Both on the internet and in person you will encounter a variety of information and personalities. Remember to take a deep breath, and tease out the quality information from that which does not serve you.

As you are exploring and taking your next steps, remember why you are exploring rope. Was it to make beautiful art? To connect with your partner in the bedroom? To experience extreme (or soft) sensations? Pause from time to time and check in with yourself and your partner and ask—are we still on a path we want to be on? If you are not, reassess, and course-correct for optimal success.

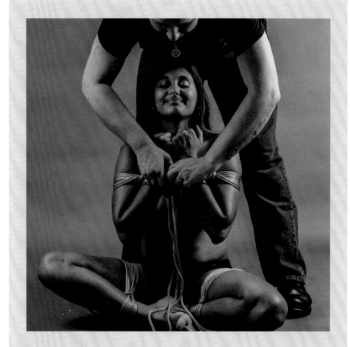

Now that you are ready to play, go ahead and choose a rope that feels good in your hand, is pleasing to your eye, and works for you and your partner.

Buy Rope!

Here are some suppliers of truly excellent rope for bondage. The list below is far from exhaustive, as new vendors are coming to the market on a regular basis, but it is a good place to start.

www.RopeExtremes.com

The beautiful MFP ropes throughout the book are examples of their work, as well as the Western hemp in the samples section.

www.BindMe.nl

Based out of the Netherlands, Marrow has been an active member of the international rope community for as long as I can remember, and provided all of the fine jute used liberally in the book.

www.AiNawa.com

Importing rope from a small production company in Japan, AiNawa also offers a wide variety of Japanese rope pornography that will inspire and titillate.

www.AjaRope.com

Aja and Lily are a homegrown business that has developed into the home of a wide variety of rope and bondage supplies, including harder to find products like hempex.

www.BastardRopes.com

These passionate rope community enthusiasts make small-batch hemp and jute rope, and have built a fantastic list of free how-to videos on their resource page.

www.BeautifulBondage.net

Home of English photographer and rigger Mark Varley, he now carries a variety of synthetic and natural ropes.

www.BossBondage.com

Purveyors of quality hemp and jute, Boss has become a well-known personality in the rope community.

www.DeGiottoRope.com

Looking for bamboo or silk rope? De Giotto is an artisan of these as well as truly silky jute rope, and a colorful variety created in-house for custom orders.

www.ErinHoudini.com

Do you want a wide variety of nylon, including vibrant UV-reactive rope? Erin Houdini is the artist and Western bondage educator for you.

www.Esinem.com

Based out of England, Esinem not only sells beautiful rope, but his site is a fantastic resource for bondage education, while he himself is also a well-known bondage educator.

www.JadeRope.com

In addition to carrying beautiful jute, hemp, cotton and linen rope, Jade Rope also sells diverse synthetic materials including "natural look" synthetics. Their resources on rope history are also well worth a visit.

www.Jakara-Rope.co.uk

Selling a variety of deluxe hemp and jute, this England-based artist has a beautiful collection of rope.

www.Jugoya.com

After years, the world-famous bondage artist Arisue Go has released his own line of Japanese bondage rope.

www.Garrs-Ropes.com

Known for their prompt and friendly service, Garr and his crew have a lovely variety of MFP rope in solid and striped colors.

www.KinkyRopes.com

Jack Elfrink has a wide selection, including flax and artificial lines like pseudo-cotton and promilla for those with allergies. His center-marked ropes help for quickly finding your bight.

www.KnotKnormal.com

Making both single-ply (Japanese style) and double-ply jute line, Knot Knormal also carries sadistic coconut rope.

www.KnottyKink.com

Based in New England, these enthusiastic artists craft bamboo, hemp and jute ropes for the beginner and expert alike.

www.M0coJute.com

With a variety of options for having your rope "finished," M0co hand-processes each rope order to your specifications.

www.RainbowRope.com

Beautiful purveyors of both artificial and natural fiber ropes, as well as a bevy of other BDSM supplies.

www.RopeSpace.com

Made by the rope artist Bodhi, this artist vends a simple selection of jute rope. In addition, this site offers free online tutorials and links to other resources.

www.ShopRopeMarks.com

Carrying beautiful red linen rope, Bob also carries jute rope in classical 8 meter lengths from Japanese bondage master Osada Steve.

www.Serenity-Bound.com

This Canadian artist sells hemp rope, but also has a great portable bondage frame they designed.

www.TwistedMonk.com

Monk's rope comes in a variety of sizes and colors, and has a great feel to it. He is the tried and true maker of rope for many erotic websites.

www.VenusRopes.com

Available in a multitude of colors, the ladies at Venus Ropes make beautiful nylon and more.

www.VintageRope.com

Artisan of fine ropes, Damon Pierce provides beautiful cotton and jute rope.

www.WitherAndDye.com

Crafting beautiful hemp rope in a wide variety of colors, these artisans are also leading the way in making suspension rings that are works of art in and of themselves.

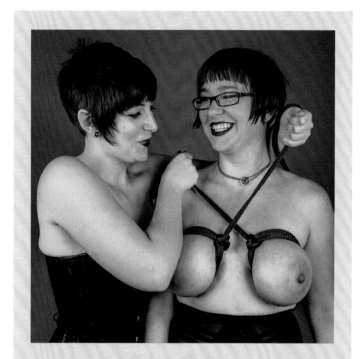

When choosing rope, make sure it is something that everyone playing will enjoy. Each vendor is unique, and some will truly make you smile.

Get Inspired by More Books

Why stop here? Here are some books that I have explored for further information on the subject of Japanese-style rope bondage, as well as other how-to books on erotic ropework. Go out and see what other folks have to say:

More Shibari You Can Use: Passionate Rope Bondage and Intimate Connection

The next in the *Shibari You Can Use* family, this book continues with this style of rope bondage, while examining why we do rope bondage as well. Techniques from upper body harnesses to head bondage, speed rope to floral knotwork ties are covered, but we also dive into power exchange, sensuality, intimacy, and emotionally journeying together in rope. Let's not look just at how to do rope, but how to connect with one another as we do it, no matter our experience level. Keep your ears open for future books in the *Shibari You Can Use* family as well.

ISBN 978-0-9778727-5-6

Bondage Basics: 52 Naughty Knots and Risqué Restraints You Need to Know

Written by Lord Morpheous (the author of *How to Be Kinky*), this book features a variety of ties and communication techniques for playing with rope. Featuring both male and female models, it is both titillating and educational.

ISBN 9781592336456

The Book of Five Rings for Rope Arts

This two-volume collection of step-by-step tutorials by Arisue Go has become a staple of modern Shibari instruction. Its break down of ties makes for clear instruction whether you speak Japanese or not. His further series *Kinbaku Mind and Techniques 1 and 2* continues with his work.

Bound: Shibari Style Impressions

David Lawrence's art book has many beautiful Japanese-style rope bondage images shot in stark black and white. He captures the essence of the beauty of Shibari and the book is a great inspiration. His follow-up books *ReBound* and *Intensity* feature further beautiful work, with Intensity featuring images of men in rope as a fundraiser for HIV/AIDS organizations.

ISBN 908077061

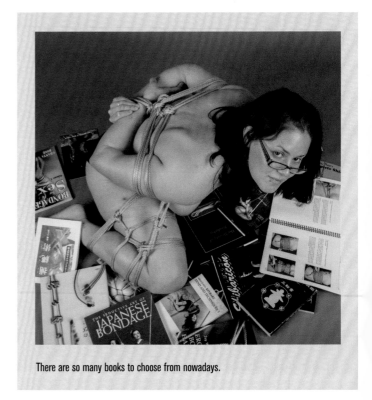
There are so many books to choose from nowadays.

Complete Shibari: Land

Douglas Kent takes a minimalist approach to his bondage book, showing images in a step-by-step manner, mirroring many Japanese-language Shibari books, which have limited text. Though many of the models can hold body positions that many of us cannot, it is a resource worth examining.

ISBN 978-0973668810

Das Bondage-Handbuch: Anleitung zum erotischen Fesseln

By Matthias T. J. Grimme, this German how-to bondage book from Black Label has many good ideas in it, and wonderful images to be inspired by.

ISBN 3-931406-16-4

The Erotic Bondage Handbook

By Jay Wiseman, this book from Greenery Press is has a lot of quality information on bondage and BDSM safety, as well as wonderful ideas on "Western" rope bondage.

ISBN 1-890159-13-1

The Essence of Shibari

This beautiful full-color book by Shin Nawakiri is the first book on Japanese rope bondage published in Chinese. Featuring both male and female models, this well-designed book shows a wide variety of ties to expand your repertoire.

ISBN 9789866474453

The Little Guide to Getting Tied Up

An insightful collection of wisdom and tools for developing your skills as a Bottom, this book by Evie Vane is a useful text for anyone and everyone who enjoys bondage. Straight-forward and conversational, it is an easy read and very accessible.

ISBN 978-1500771683

Pleasure in the Fall

By Minako Ogawa, a.k.a. Daraku, this book from Japan Mix Inc. is one of the most elegant art books presenting Japanese bondage available on the market today.

ISBN 4-88321-475-3

Rope, Bondage and Power

It was my absolute honor to edit this anthology of 20 rope bondage enthusiasts and educators from around the world. Instead of diving into how to do bondage, it explores why we do rope bondage. From Zen approaches to hot pornographic memories, women and men, Tops and Bottoms, novices and life-long explorers all share their journeys and unique perspectives.

ISBN 978-1935509028

Rope for Sex – Volume 1

This beautiful collection of erotic step-by-step ties by Chanta Rose is a wonderful way to get turned on. The porn models throughout the book show a variety of poses for the lithe and active to get going in the bedroom.

ISBN 978-0977723805

The Seductive Art of Japanese Bondage

Written by Midori and photographed by Craig Morey, this book is an outstanding source for excellent tutorials and the history of Japanese rope bondage.

ISBN 1-890159-38-7

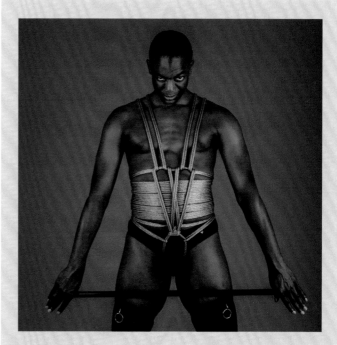

A short Rope Corset (page 86) can create quite the dapper, or villainous, look.

Shibari: The Art of Japanese Bondage

Master "K" has a distinct eye for capturing Shibari on film, and his lovely informational book on the subject gives some great ideas of what can be done with this art form. His further book, *The Beauty of Kinbaku*, is an invaluable resource on the history of Shibari.

ISBN 978908770620

Showing You the Ropes

In clear and concise text with images, the Two Knotty Boys share their approach to fusion bondage. Almost all of the ties can be easily modified (or are shown) for a wide variety of bodies, and feature beautiful knotwork broken down into easy-to-follow steps. Their sequel, *Back on the Ropes*, stands alone or can be used together with their other book, and both complement the work in the *Shibari You Can Use* books.

ISBN 978-1931160490

Getting Inspired by Other People's Bondage

There are so many amazing rope artists doing work worldwide. Ten years ago, there were very few ways to find each other or see each other's work, but nowadays by typing "Japanese rope bondage" into a search engine, you can find a lot. Mind you, some is excellent, and some is less so. I am listing below some of my favorite places to find inspiration from other people's ropework.

www.FetLife.com

A kink community social networking site, FetLife features thousands of discussion groups, including a large number on rope bondage. I recommend starting with "Riggers and Rope Sluts" (group 51), "Shibari" (group 195) and "Adult Rope Art" (group 2816). The Adult Rope Art group is a continuation of the group founded in the late '90s, and is full of links and resources for exploring not only rope bondage, but the rope bondage community as well. Think twice about putting up images of yourself before you do so—once something is on the internet, it might just stay on the internet. FetLife also features an image "love" function, and the "Kinky and Popular" area often features truly inspirational rope bondage photography. If you are new to exploring the kink or rope communities online or in person, consider getting a copy of *Playing Well With Others: Your Guide to Discovering, Exploring and Navigating the BDSM, Kink and Leather Communities* by Lee Harrington and Mollena Williams.

www.FusionKnots.com

Though it is not a BDSM site, Fusion Knots is a great place to learn new knots, and get lots of inspiration for making truly beautiful artwork on your partner's body.

www.JapaneseRopeArt.com

Hosted by Master Tatu of Florida, this website has a large amount of written information on Japanese rope bondage that is worth consideration.

www.Kinbaku-Art.com

Zamil has a unique and beautiful vision for rope bondage that shows through in performances, photography and education.

www.KinbakuLuxuria.com

Riccardo Sergnese (aka Wildties) is a rope artist out of Italy, who has an eye for the beauty of Japanese aesthetic bondage. His website features a variety of images to tantalize and inspire.

www.Kink.com

One of the top pornography companies internationally, Kink.com has excelled in BDSM imagery in part because they have brought on some of the top riggers in the world to do the bondage on their site. They also regularly hire models whose athleticism makes them capable of doing poses that the average person cannot even consider doing. They have trained up to the level of the extreme sports they engage in, and just like few of us can run a marathon (even with training), so it is for many of the ties shown. Their sites provide intense inspiration for directions you may want to evolve your own art, from visual details to role-playing possibilities.

www.Kybari.com

One of the top artisans in the world of "rope fashion," Fred Kryel's bondage is a thing of beauty and inspiration alike. Having learned how to tie rope corsets and chest harnesses in this book, you can see in Kryel's work where the next steps in erotic macramé can lead.

www.LordMorpheous.com

Author, rigger and photographer, Lord Morpheous is also the producer for "Morpheous' Bondage Extravaganza" in Toronto. With over 100 performers from around the world, running from dusk to dawn, it has become an international phenomenon.

www.NawaPedia.com

This simply designed resource listing includes a wide variety of kinbaku, shibari and asian aesthetic rope artists from around the globe.

www.OsadaSteve.com

Nawashi Osada Steve is one of the premier Japanese bondage artists today, and his how-to videos and astounding performances are a must-see for individuals who want to continue with more traditional Shibari. He has founded the Osada Ryu (Osada-Ryu.com) school of Shibari, which has a formal lineage of training to perfect not only the katas (techniques and patterns) of Japanese bondage, but also the energy and connection.

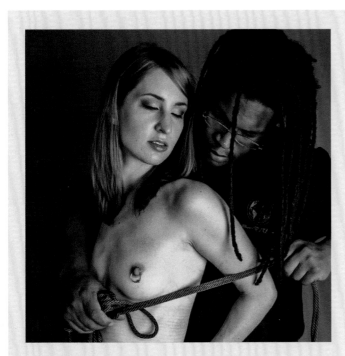
You don't always need complex ties. One piece of rope can do a whole lot.

www.RemedialRopes.com

An amazing resource for rope Bottoms and Tops alike, Stefanos and Shay have brought together a wide variety of essays in one location. From basic bondage safety to understanding nerve damage, rope myths to developing confidence, and this site is a must-see for everyone into rope.

www.RopeCast.com

This podcast by Graydancer is the longest running podcast on rope bondage online. With interviews, features on bondage events, and an intimate view on the GRUE (Greydancer's Ropetastic Unconference Extravaganza), the RopeCast is a fantastic place to get inspired.

www.RopeMarks.com

Bob is an amazing rigger and performance artist from Amsterdam, whose creativity is ever evolving and worth checking in on from time to time.

www.Shibaricon.com

Shibaricon is a massive rope bondage conference that takes place yearly in Chicago, Illinois, bringing together rope bondage students, players, teachers and performers from around the world. Getting inspired in person, as well as learning from others in the flesh, is a fantastic way to evolve your rope exploration. Other rope bondage conferences now exist around the globe, ranging in size, level of expertise, and venue. Look for one in your area, or consider making a vacation out of investing in your erotic evolution.

www.Vimeo.com

The home for a wide variety of beautiful videos of all forms, type "kinbaku" or "shibari" into the search engine to find inspiring performances and educational opportunities.

There are also a variety of places on the internet to go explore tutorials after getting the basics of the ties in this book under your belt. They include:

- www.BDSM-Chicago.com/cram
- www.BeKnotty.com
- www.Encordees.com
- www.KinkAcademy.com
- www.KinkUniversity.com
- www.Kikkou.com
- www.MassachusettsBondage.com
- www.MonkeyFetish.com
- www.NaturallyTwisted.co
- www.Rope-Topia.com
- www.RopeFashions.com
- www.Shibari-By.com
- www.TwistedMonk.com
- www.TwoKnottyBoys.com

Practice, Practice, Practice!

That's right: no matter how much you read or stare at pretty pictures, you won't really get a feel for shibari until you start doing it yourself. Practice on friends or your own ankle. Keep a pile of rope in a drawer next to the bed for a bit of fun. Go to parties. Find workshops to attend. Consider going to a BDSM or bondage conference.

Slip this book into the hands of your partner and say, "Hey, wanna try, just once?"

And if what you have found out is that you like crotch ropes and the rest is not for you? Awesome. Your next right step might be to set down this book, and head to the bedroom right now to keep "practicing" that tie with enthusiasm and a big smile.

Have fun, be authentically you, and enjoy the rope techniques you have learned. You now have in your hands, shibari you can use!

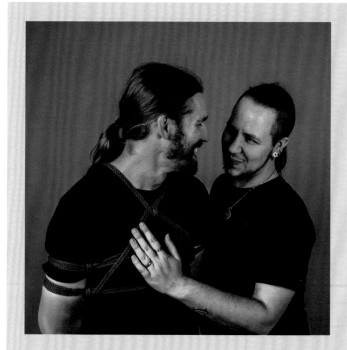

Play responsibly, and remember to have fun!

Acknowledgements

A lot has happened since 2004 when the creation of Shibari You Can Use began. But here we are, a decade later, and I am so honored that the project has turned into a beloved staple of the rope bondage community and beyond. But it was time for a facelift, this time in full color. The book shows most of the same step-by-step ties it did before, but has been re-shot with new models and the text has been clarified using the feedback from readers and fans over the years. In addition, the listing of bondage resources has been updated and expanded to reflect the ever-growing world of rope.

Thanks go out to my partners and family of the heart who have put up with me during the creation of this book in all of its incarnations. Disappearing for days at a time to go teach at universities and sexuality conferences is one thing, but holing up in my office when I am home, or heading out to hide and write is another. You have been such a blessing.

In the original production of the book I was blessed through working with the amazing Circle23, and finding someone to step into his shoes for the second edition seemed like it might be challenging.

I was grateful to be wrong. RiggerJay has proven himself to not only be a fantastic photographer and adventure partner, but friend and supporter who has the guts to lovingly kick me in the ass from time to time. I literally could not have done this without him. The hours, heart, and passion he has poured into this book are mind-blowing, and I am grateful for all that he has done and is as a person.

It is hard enough to model for an original project, but can be even more so when re-shooting images that need replicated while bringing a fresh energy. I am so grateful for my amazing models on the Second Edition: Amy Morgan, Ay, Ayem Willing, Barracudabite, BendYogaGirl, Calico, Deanna Cannonball, Ginger Baker, Jester35, Just Derek, Klawdya Rothschild, Knave Karina, Lily Ligotage, Mecha Kate, Miss Seraph, Mollena Williams, Murphy Blue, Naked Amanda, Nayland Blake, Nightshades, Scotty Thomson, Spiral, Walkyrie, and Yandy.

Ayem Willing (the last model shown in the book with an amazing smile on his face) was also an amazing advocate for this project... and friend. He will be missed as he journeys to the rope suspension rig beyond the veil.

Thank you as well to my original models who created the framework from which we were able to craft this work. Alone in Darkness, Astrid, Becca, Black Dove, Duncan, Desiree Wolfe, Evie (slave62), Jaguar, Kitten, Lauren, Lusid, Peach, Reverend 7, and Yasmin Ling—you were an amazing team to collaborate with.

On the shoots this time around we also had a number of fantastic assistant riggers: JustDerek, Murphy Blue, and Bill from RopeExtremes. Your aid kept the ropes flying, making both models and myself so grateful.

In the past two versions of the book my crew of editors also helped make some magic that led eventually to this version: DaliGraphics, Scott C. Brown and Audrey Eschright. For copy editing in this edition, the much-appreciated amazing eyes and feedback of Roxy (perfectly_bound) and Nannette H. were invaluable. Rob River has been with me for two versions of this book now, crafting the beautiful covers for this edition and the last, as well as stepping in to do the interior layout on the print version of the revised edition as well. Rob, you have been truly amazing, on so many fronts. Paul Petrie and his printing crew whisked in with amazing ideas and paper vision to bring the project into a classy light while making me smile. And of course the folks at IPG were an amazing whirlwind resource on so many levels that I am grateful for.

We could not have done this project without the fantastic venues involved. RiggerJay, your place helped make so much magic and fun possible, not just for your photo studio, but for the kitchen floor that was crawled on. KLAWTEX at the House of Yes, thank you for allowing us use of your spaces for shooting in Brooklyn. Cauldron Farm and Hartley House, thank you for all of your support with the first versions of the book, providing a place away from the world to pour out my heart while you fed me. To Catherynne M. Valente and Dmitri, thank you for opening up your magical writing retreat space in Maine to this road-weary traveler. And to my Ramblewood tribe, Harry Leff, Kalabran Friedel, James, Jamie and Danny... you never cease to make me feel welcomed, even a decade later.

I can only hope that my rope work and teaching reflects as proudly on my teachers as their spirit and art has touched and inspired me. But having been in the public kink communities since 1996, it seems that many of my rope teachers have become friends; teachers have become students, students have become teachers, and friends and siblings in rope have continued to inspire and teach me every day. These include, but are not limited to: Aiden Fyre, Artemis, Bob from RopeMarks, Boss Bondage, Cannon, Claire Adams, Coral Mallow, Delano N. Distress, Dov H., Eddie, Emma Hui, Esinem, Graydancer, Hedwig, Ice, James Mogul, Janice Stine, Joel Albert (and his teacher Lou Duff), Juliet Heart, Karri, Lenora, Lochai, Lolita and Philip Wolf, LqqkOut, LthrEdge, Madame Butterfly, Madison Young, Mark, Aleni, and Lani of House Dv8, Master "K," Max of Seattle, Mick and Dee Luvbight, Midori, MorTis, MRK, Murphy and Diamond Blue, Neptune Glory, Paul Bates, Peter Slemrian, Saki Kamijoo, Scott Smith, Sir C, Stella Perversa, Stickman, SxySadist Suzanne, Tifereth, Tom Wood, Twisted Monk, and Zamil. Special love and memory goes out to Maria Shadoes, model and friend alike.

Three people very close to me kept me on course in the final legs of this project. Mitch Beyer was my guiding light of fetish missionary work, who reminded me that the world deserves erotic adventure, and that I could be that voice. J.D. of Two Knotty Boys kicked me in the ass while providing me with insight, philosophy, wisdom, a home away from home, and a mirror of knotted passion. And Butterfly gave me space to be myself while inspiring me to do ever better in both love and life. Beyond these three amazing humans, I remain eternally grateful to Bear, for all of the opportunities I have been granted to serve.

Last but not least, the folks I could never have made it this far without: my fans and students. Thank you for having faith in me and pestering me regularly in person, on email and on various social media sites to make the Revised Edition of the project happen. Special thanks go out to every single one of the Indiegogo supporters who have brought this project to light. Your communication with me—between private emails, in-person conversations and photos of how you've made this work your own... you make it all worth it.

Yours in Passion and Soul,

Lee Harrington
Anchorage, Alaska, USA
December 2014

About the Author

Lee Harrington is an internationally known spiritual and erotic authenticity educator, gender explorer, eclectic artist and award-winning author and editor on human erotic and sacred experience. He is a nice guy with a disarmingly down to earth approach to the fact that we are each beautifully complex ecosystems, and we deserve to examine the human experience from that lens. He's been traveling the globe (from Seattle to Sydney, Berlin to Boston), teaching and talking about sexuality, psychology, faith, desire and more, and is grateful for the journeys and love he has found along the way. He has been an academic and a female adult film performer, a world-class sexual adventurer, a published fetish photographer, an outspoken philosopher, a kink/bondage expert, and has been blogging about sex and spirituality since 1998.

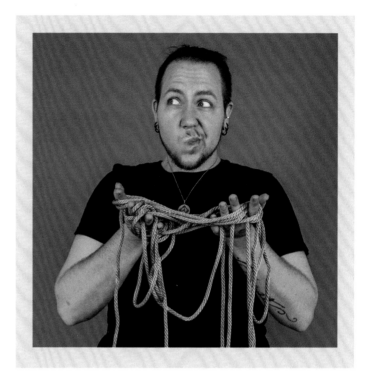

His books include *More Shibari You Can Use: Passionate Rope Bondage and Intimate Connection, Playing Well With Others: Your Guide to Discovering, Exploring and Negotiating the Kink, Leather and BDSM Communities* (with Mollena Williams), *Sacred Kink: The Eightfold Paths of BDSM and Beyond, Shibari You Can Use: Japanese Rope Bondage and Erotic Macramé,* the *Toybag Guide to Age Play, On Starry Thighs: Sacred and Sensual Poetry,* and *Shed Skins: Journeying in Self-Portraits.* He has also worked as an anthology editor on such projects as *Rope, Bondage, and Power* and *Spirit of Desire: Personal Explorations of Sacred Kink,* while contributing actively to other anthologies, magazines, blogs, and collaborations.

Check out the trouble Lee has been getting into, as well as his regular podcast, tour schedule, free essays, videos, coaching, and more at www.PassionAndSoul.com.

About the Photographer

By RopeRaiden and Twisted Phoenix

We first met RiggerJay online when he emailed us asking us a bunch of great questions about our ties and pictures. He came out to Detroit in fall of 2007 to take pictures of us and learn for the weekend. This was his first experience seeing Shibari-inspired suspension and from there he became a student of Japanese-inspired rope bondage. The pictures he took of us that weekend are still some of our most treasured pictures ever taken! Needless to say, a very close and dear friendship has transpired.

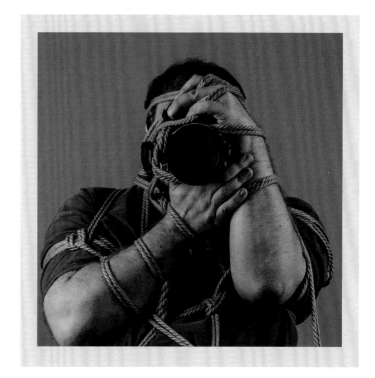

After this first meeting, we told him to attend Shibaricon with us to experience even more. It was at this event RiggerJay met Lee Harrington. Eventually, he would take private lessons with Lee and they became friends. This inspired RiggerJay to use his photography skills to capture the intimacy and artistry of Shibari in all its forms. He finds the intertwining of the artistry and technical aspects of both rope and photography fascinating and fulfilling.

One of the most interesting connections about this collaboration between RiggerJay and Lee is that the original book, *Shibari You Can Use* was the first book Rigger Jay ever bought on the subject of Shibari, it was in his hands when we first met him. In 2013, RiggerJay's skill and passion were used to re-shoot the pictures for the revised version of that same book. Now, his photography is in book two of this series as well.

RiggerJay can be found today sharing his rope and photography skills at many different events in the US and Canada. Centered in New England, his efforts have led to many rope groups forming and spreading his philosophy of "Watch—Read—Learn, then make it your own."

You can see more of RiggerJay's work at **www.RiggerJay.com** and **RiggerJay.tumblr.com**.